Healing the Female Heart

For decades, women's hearts have been ignored while men's have been analyzed and cared for. Yet 247,000 women die every year from heart attacks. *It doesn't have to be this way.* Whether you are old or young, have been diagnosed with heart disease or are in good health, you have the power to protect your own heart. Starting today, you can learn:

- How to weigh your risk factors for heart disease, and what to do to reduce them.
- How to develop an exercise and nutrition program that works for you.
- How to handle stress and develop the inner peace that will strengthen your heart.
- How to make sure your doctor asks for the right tests to properly diagnose a heart condition.
- How to weigh the risks and benefits of hormone replacement therapy, and decide if it's right for you.
- How to get the very best care in the emergency room.
- How to prepare yourself, mentally and physically, for heart surgery.
- How to survive a heart attack and recuperate fully—both physically and emotionally.
- How to reclaim your sexuality, without fear, after a heart attack.

Healing the Female Heart

A HOLISTIC APPROACH TO PREVENTION AND RECOVERY FROM HEART DISEASE

Elizabeth Ross, M.D.,

AND

Judith Sachs

A LYNN SONBERG BOOK

POCKET BOOKS

New York   London   Toronto   Sydney   Tokyo   Singapore

Research about heart disease and hormone replacement therapy is ongoing and subject to interpretation. Although efforts have been made to include the most up-to-date and accurate information in this book, there can be no guarantee that what we know about this complex subject won't change with time. Readers should bear in mind that this book should not be used for self-diagnosis or self-treatment and should consult their physicians regarding all health issues. The author and publisher disclaim any liability arising directly or indirectly from the use of this book.

An *Original* Publication of POCKET BOOKS

POCKET BOOKS, a division of Simon & Schuster Inc.
1230 Avenue of the Americas, New York, NY 10020

Published by arrangement with Lynn Sonberg Book Associates,
10 West 86 Street, New York, NY 10024

Library of Congress Cataloging-in-Publication Data

Ross, Elizabeth, M.D.
    Healing the female heart : a holistic approach to prevention and
recovery from heart disease / Elizabeth Ross and Judith Sachs.
        p. cm.
    "A Lynn Sonberg book."
    Includes index.
    ISBN: 0-671-89470-6
    1. Heart—Diseases. 2. Women—Diseases. 3. Heart—Diseases—
Prevention. I. Sachs, Judith, 1947– . II. Title.
RC682.R675 1996
616.1′2′0082—dc20   95-9494
                                                                 CIP

First Pocket Books trade paperback printing January 1996

10 9 8 7 6 5 4 3 2 1

POCKET and colophon are registered trademarks of
Simon & Schuster Inc.

Printed in the U.S.A.

For my Grandmother Isabel Sieber,
a suffragette
who taught me
to be a critical thinker.

E.R.

For Dr. Hensley,
whose great heart
has helped me
to keep the beat.

J.S.

Acknowledgments

The authors are deeply grateful to many individuals who freely gave their time and energy to help in the preparation of this book. We would like to thank Fred Weinberg, M.D., and his patients; Dean Ornish, M.D.; Bonnie Arkus and the Queen of Hearts; Pat McGovern, R.N., and the staff of St. Francis Rehabilitation Center; Ken Lee, M.D., and the team at Washington Heart who so graciously allowed Judith Sachs to observe cardiac procedures; the Jersey Shore Medical Center; and Dr. Wulf Utian and the North American Menopause Society.

Contents

Preface

When I first started my practice in cardiology, I was at first puzzled and then dumbfounded at the number of women I saw who had serious heart disease. I had finished my medical training with the misconception that women were protected from this disease, which is a major killer of American men. As I quietly went about the task of reeducating myself, I was astonished to learn that coronary heart disease is also the major killer of American women. Six times as many women die from heart attacks as die from breast cancer every year in the United States; the number of women who will die from heart attacks is also greater than the number of those who will die from all forms of cancer in women combined.

I began volunteering for the American Heart Association, and I became committed to raising everyone's awareness of the magnitude of this problem. I gave lectures to women's groups, at churches and synagogues, and I discussed the issue on local television and radio programs. Mostly everyone I spoke with— patients, physicians, nurses and therapists—also believed that heart attacks only affected men. One episode I vividly remember occurred during a cocktail party when a woman asked me what I did for a living. I replied that I took care of women with heart problems.

She answered coyly, "Oh, you're a psychiatrist."

I was speechless but not entirely surprised. I have seen countless patients with serious heart disease who were told they were just anxious or depressed, and others who have had symptoms that they brushed off as indigestion or fatigue.

From 1983 to 1988, I completed two fellowships (one in cardiac pathology at the National Institutes of Health, one in cardiology at Washington Hospital Center), and here I began to see increasing numbers of female patients with heart disease. I have now been in clinical practice for thirteen years and worked on the committee on women and heart disease of the Washington chapter of the American Heart Association. During this time, I have cared for hundreds of women in various stages of heart disease and have therefore had a unique view of this illness—from the inside out. I felt that I had a mission to write this book, in collaboration with Judith Sachs, because I needed to tell more women about the dangers of ignoring their hearts, and the positive results of adopting a preventive lifestyle.

I have had the privilege and sorrow of obtaining a close-up view of our greatest national tragedy. In the United States, nearly one quarter of a million deaths from heart attack occur to women each year.

So why do we still think of heart disease as a man's problem? In truth, the prevalence of heart disease has been decreasing for men since the 1950s while it has steadily increased for women.

When a man complains of chest pain, he gets a treadmill exercise test. When a woman complains of chest pain, she may be given medicines and a gentle reassurance that the discomfort is "just nerves" or menopause or empty-nest syndrome. Few women have an exercise test as part of an executive physical, though it is a routine procedure for men over forty. Men tend to show symptoms of heart disease in their late forties and early fifties, but women don't exhibit these symptoms until after menopause. At this point, when they are fifty-five to sixty-five years old, they are as likely to have heart disease as men. Because they live typically eight to ten years longer than their male companions, this gives them the potential for decades of disability resulting from heart disease.

What makes the female heart work? What makes it break down? Experts are certain that blood lipid levels and female hormones play large roles, as do risk factors like cigarette smoking, high blood pressure, diabetes, and family history. Personality and the inability to handle stress seem to have an ever-increasing influence, as we discover how intricately mind and body are linked to keep us healthy or allow us to become ill.

Despite the overwhelming evidence that proper treatment of risk factors has a significant impact on future health, many women are inadequately screened for the risk factors that contribute to heart disease. I have seen women with cholesterol levels of more than 300 who have been told by their physicians not to worry because women don't get heart attacks.

But they do, and the numbers are increasing. If a woman has a heart attack, she is twice as likely to die in the first year after the attack as a man. In addition, it usually takes twice as much time after a heart attack for a woman to be referred to a major cardiac center for further evaluation and treatment. And some physicians defend their less-than-aggressive treatment, stating that since women have higher complication and death rates following procedures like cardiac catheterization, balloon angioplasty, and coronary bypass surgery, it's safer to take a wait-and-see course of action.

But analysis of the data about *why* women do poorly in these procedures reveals the truth: by the time they are referred for treatment, they are older and sicker and have more advanced stages of heart disease as well as coexistent medical problems such as diabetes or osteoporosis. One of the reasons for this is that the female heart is more difficult to fathom than the male heart—and until very recently, the medical establishment was populated primarily by men, who were working hard on the problems of male heart disease.

Men, rather than women, were those used in clinical trials for the benefits and drawbacks of all the medications indicated for the treatment of heart disease. The surgical instruments designed for heart surgery were built for men's larger hearts; procedures such as angiography, angioplasty, and bypass surgery were performed on men. Many clinical trials conducted on men have shown that a daily aspirin is effective for men as a preventive measure to thin the blood and prevent clots. Will it work for women as well as it does for men? One large study on a group of nurses indicates that the answer is yes, but we won't know definitively until more women-only clinical trials take place.

And as researchers leapt ahead with male-centered improvements in heart disease treatment, women sickened and suffered silently.

Why? Because a woman very often has no idea that her heart is not functioning properly until it's too late. Her entire life may center around taking care of others, ignoring her own pain, refusing to see the doctor until her spouse, her parents, and her children have been diagnosed, treated, and cared for. What's a twinge across the chest every once in a while, even if the twinges go on for ten years? They're uncomfortable, that's all. And for so many women with heart disease, there's no twinge at all.

Healing the Female Heart explains the urgency of being informed and taking action on your own behalf. It is essential that each woman understand her risk factors and get the proper screening and evaluation for her condition.

A woman can do a lot, just in terms of changing her lifestyle. She can lose weight if she is overweight, stop smoking, get treatment for her high blood pressure, lower her cholesterol, manage her stress more effectively, and maintain a regular exercise regimen that will protect her heart. And she can work closely in coordination with her health-care professional to get the kind of treatment she needs, whether it be medication or surgery.

A great deal of progress has been made in cardiac care in the past few years, and the more we know about what can be done, the better equipped we will be to combat this killer. Each woman can benefit from this healing course, whether she has been diagnosed with heart disease or just wants to improve her future heart health.

How This Book Can Help

If every woman reading this book learns what she has to do to stay well, how she can determine if she's at risk, and what to do if she becomes ill, she can beat the odds on women's heart disease. The following chapters explain how a woman's heart works, the common risk factors for heart disease, and how to follow a good preventive health-care plan. Then we'll take you through the various problems that might occur—from coronary artery disease to mitral valve prolapse to silent ischemia to Syndrome X. We'll explain all the various tests that should be done to confirm a diagnosis of heart disease and will outline a sensible plan of diet, exercise, medication, and surgery that will help you stay healthy despite your heart condition. Another chapter will cover ways to minimize damage after a heart attack, and finally, we will address some very profound issues that will make you question some ingrained attitudes about what you want for the rest of your life. Where to Go for Help, at the back of the book, will direct you to organizations and support groups you will need on your journey to better heart health.

You hold the reins of your health care—and your future. It is going to require some work, and you'll have to join forces with an informed medical professional in order to get a personalized plan of what you need to do, but that's not a high price to pay for a healthy future. Armed with up-to-date information on holistic prevention, early detection, and appropriate treatment, every woman can learn how to work with her physician for the best possible care.

We've handed all the responsibility for our health care over to doctors and research scientists, and for too many years, most of us have remained in the dark about what *we* have to do ourselves. Now it's time to establish a new balance of power.

Be aware! Your heart is your most prized possession. Whether you are currently concerned about heart disease or you never thought about it before, whether you are reading this book for your mother, your sister, or yourself—it is time to consider new ways to protect the cardiovascular system.

—Elizabeth Ross, M.D., F.A.C.C.
Fellow of the American College of Cardiology

Healing the
Female Heart

1

The Female Heart
Is More Than a Valentine

∇

Marcia didn't usually take time out of her incredibly hectic day to go to her husband's doctor's appointment, but it was a week away from Bob's fiftieth birthday, which they both felt was a significant milestone. He'd been fine since the mild heart attack he'd suffered five years ago, but he still sometimes said that he thought he was living on borrowed time. Since she was six years older than he was, and women typically outlive their husbands by just that much, they always joked that they could die happily together.

Marcia sat beside Bob in the consultation room and listened as the doctor told her everything she was going to do to keep Bob just as healthy as he was for another ten years.

"Marcia, I want you to make sure this guy gets out and walks two miles a day or does something to move his carcass around, all right?"

"*I'm* supposed to make him exercise!" she laughed, thinking that the two of them were inveterate couch potatoes. Bob only exercised under duress, and she never did.

"And you know all about low-cholesterol cooking by now, I hope," the doctor continued. "No eggs, no butter, no—"

"No nothing yummy," Marcia concluded. "We're sort of all right about that, except when Bob cooks, and then heaven help our arteries."

"Hey," Bob interjected, "what about that fish swimming in cream sauce you served the other night? And the beef stroganoff we had the night before that?"

"Well, yes," Marcia confessed. "True." Why did she suddenly feel guilty about making him what he'd asked for?

"How about the smoking?" asked the doctor. "Are you keeping him away from cigarettes?"

"He's quit, but I haven't," Marcia said truthfully. "I just don't know how to do it. I've tried so many programs, and I've tried to do it on my own, but no success. I guess I don't have much willpower. He's better about that than I am—I hope it'll rub off."

The doctor shook a finger at her. "It better, or you'll get him angry. And we don't want his stress level going up, so keep things on an even keel between the two of you, will you, Marcia?"

Bob smiled. "It's not Marcia, it's the job that stresses me out. But I couldn't function if I wasn't challenged by my work," Bob claimed. "I thrive on it. She's the one you should talk to about controlling her anger. She's got this boss who won't let her get a word in edgewise, keeps her late, makes her take stuff home—it's lousy."

"Sorry about that. Now, Bob," the doctor concluded, "I'll call when we get the lab results of your HDL and LDL cholesterol and your blood sugar, but the ECG and treadmill test look good, which means that so far you've got a clean bill of health. Anything else you folks want to tell me?"

Marcia stared at their doctor, trying to remember the last time she'd been in here for a checkup—she did visit her gynecologist once a year, but it had been a long time since she'd seen their family doctor for a complete exam. Could it have been five years ago, when Bob was sick? She remembered sitting in this same chair then, saying something about her own father's heart attack. He'd had a major infarction that killed him when he was forty-five, and because Bob was the same age when he had his mild attack, the event had really terrified her. The past seemed to be coming back to haunt her.

"So how're you doing, Marcia?" the doctor asked as he led them to the door.

"Just fine, thanks," she murmured. As she walked into the waiting room, another pang hit her chest. She was having these weird gas pains a lot lately. But they stopped as soon as she sat down and rested, so she'd never mentioned them to anyone.

"I guess I should come in for a checkup," Marcia said to Bob as they walked to the front desk to pay the bill.

Bob glanced down at the list of charges. "I don't know if we could afford for both of us to have this exam," he muttered.

But Marcia can't afford to go on like this, either. It could cost her her life.

The Pace of a Woman's Life—A Deciding Factor in Her Health

Marcia's situation, unfortunately, is too common. A woman of fifty-six, concerned about her husband, who has had a cardiac event in the past, is attentive to everything the doctor says about her spouse's heart health, completely ignoring the fact that *she is more at risk than he is.*

Marcia is aware of her family history, yet she hasn't had a checkup in five years. She doesn't like to think about the "gas pains" she's experiencing periodically and hasn't even told her husband and doctor about them. The smoking, the poor eating habits, and the lack of exercise are catching up with her, but does she make an attempt to change, to help herself? She seems to feel so many other things are more important. Yet nothing in the world is as important as her heart!

As in Marcia's case, we tend to neglect the one individual in our lives who really needs some nurturing—ourselves. And that omission will come back to haunt us in later life, when we cannot repair the damage of countless days and nights of self-sacrifice, stress, improper health habits, and an inability to see ourselves and our lives in perspective.

Let us analyze the scene above and shed some light on Marcia's precarious position:

- She is fifty-six, just past menopause. She no longer has the protective effect of estrogen on her heart that she had during her reproductive years because her body has drastically cut back on its hormonal production.
- She is a smoker.
- She doesn't exercise.
- She has stress on her job.
- Her eating patterns are erratic—she and her husband apparently have trouble maintaining a low-fat, low-cholesterol diet.
- She hasn't had a checkup in five years.
- The final and perhaps most significant risk factor for Marcia is that her father died of a heart attack when he was forty-five.

If you are anything like Marcia, you are not paying enough attention to yourself. You may be too busy caring for others to think about your own situation. You may skip meals or eat junk food on the run, avoid making time for exercise programs, and throw yourself into chores and activities that may strain your physical and emotional resources to the maximum.

You may not even know what your risks are. If you're a smoker, if you have hypertension, if you are diabetic, if you have elevated cholesterol, or if you have a family history that would predispose you to heart disease, it's time to get examined by a professional and make some important lifestyle changes.

When you begin to take stock of your health, the first things you must concentrate on are diet, exercise, and the factors just mentioned above. And the next factor on the list that you must attend to is stress.

How's your worry quotient? Does every tiny detail cause your gut to churn, your head to pound? Do you have any idea how to relax? Think about your own responses to emotional events that hit you during the day. Do you prioritize your issues, or does each one carry the same weight for you? Because women play so many roles in their lives, they often load one responsibility on top of another and insist that they can handle them all. Women tend to deal poorly with stress and often cover their inability to cope with excesses of other kinds, like going without sleep, smoking cigarettes, or abusing alcohol or recreational drugs.

Every factor tallies up over the years. In your thirties or forties, you may be able to function perfectly well with occasional shortness of breath, tingling in the arm, or heaviness in the chest. But the damage done over the decades may show up dramatically in your fifties and sixties. Around the time of menopause, when the female body loses the protective benefit offered by the gonadal hormone, estrogen, many women are finally diagnosed with heart disease.

Marcia is playing fast and loose with her health. Although the crisis may not hit her this week or even next year, if she continues to neglect her health care and ignore her risk factors, she may in fact be headed for a serious bout with heart disease—even a heart attack.

She could make so many important but simple changes in her daily routine that would save her life—from what she eats to how she deals with her husband to the types of mental and emotional benefits she offers herself—changes that would actually alter her destiny.

Heart disease doesn't have to strike every woman who has a complex, multilayered life. But even if heart disease has struck already, it can in many cases be successfully reversed. We all have the power to protect ourselves throughout our life span. But it will take some doing—and that is the goal of this book. By alerting yourself to the really important issues and downplaying those that are out of your control, you can set yourself on the road to having a healthier heart.

It Is Time to Pay Attention to Women's Heart Disease

Although heart disease typically strikes women ten to fifteen years later than men, it hits them hard. Although fewer women than men experience a heart attack as their first symptom of coronary disease, those who do are twice as likely as men to die after their first heart attack and two times more likely than men to have a second attack. And if they do survive, they may subsequently succumb to a second attack or a stroke. Their chances of dying after coronary bypass surgery are twice that of men, and they have lower success rates from treatments such as balloon angioplasty.

Amazingly, the above information has been downplayed and even denied by many women and the medical establishment that serves them.

Women are not the same as men. Biologically, physiologically, and emotionally, we have many unique characteristics that set us apart. Now that we are becoming aware of our special health-care needs, we are no longer content to be ignored or ridiculed for our symptoms and conditions. We will not accept second-rate, sometimes patronizing treatment for our problems. As more and more women seize control of their well-being and ask for a legitimate partnership in care with their health-care provider, the need for up-to-date, accessible information about women's health issues becomes even more essential.

Here are the facts:

• Heart disease is the number-one killer of women, accounting for approximately 247,000 of the 520,000 heart-attack deaths in our country each year. If you count deaths from all heart and blood vessel diseases combined, the tally mounts to 500,000 women's lives each year. Women are six times more likely to die from heart disease than from breast cancer and twice as likely to die from stroke as from lung cancer.

• One-third of all heart attacks among women are never reported to physicians. There are two reasons for this: either the

attacks are silent—without symptoms—and the women themselves don't know that they've had an attack; or, although the
attacks are excruciatingly painful, the women deny that anything
out of the ordinary has taken place and just accept the pain.
They don't realize that they are doing even more damage to their
hearts by not getting treatment.

• Heart disease is simply not the same in men and women.
The disease develops differently in women, and there are a
host of biological differences between the sexes and also vast
differences in the size of body organs and tissues.

• Women react very differently from men to stress, which
affects the heart.

• Hypertension is a more significant risk factor for women than
men. Women with high blood pressure are nearly four times
more likely to have heart disease as those with normal pressure,
as opposed to men, who are three times more likely.

• Even when appropriate diagnosis and treatment are begun,
the outcomes are chancier for women, largely because the existing diagnostic and surgical technology was designed by men for
men. For example, both coronary bypass surgery and balloon
angioplasty are less successful when performed on women. Current drug treatments are also less effective for women than
for men.

Why has medical science lagged so far behind in detecting and
treating women's heart disease? Why haven't women been aware
of their risks and demanded appropriate care? The reasons are
many and stem from the various "missed beats" over the years
in the research and treatment of heart disease in general. Let's
look at the history of this process.

Discrimination in Health Care for Women's Heart Disease

For decades, our hearts have been ignored while men's hearts
have been analyzed and cared for. Female heart disease is most
often manifested by years of angina (chest pain) that may be

ignored by both patient and physician. The disease takes much longer to develop in a woman, so by the time she arrives in a doctor's office for her first diagnosis she may be much sicker than a man who shows up in the emergency room with a heart attack. There are so many factors involved in the neglect of women's heart disease as an urgent health issue. Let's examine some of them.

INADEQUATE DIAGNOSIS

Women are far less likely to get an early diagnosis of heart disease. And the longer they are sick, the more severe their condition by the time it is finally detected. Dr. Bernadine Healy, former head of the National Institutes of Health, called this sex bias in treatment "the Yentl syndrome," after the story by I. B. Singer. Just as Yentl had to pretend she was a boy in order to become educated, so women with coronary heart disease have had to suffer a major heart attack before doctors would take their condition seriously. It sounds impossible, but a case like Shirley Applebaum's is all too common.

Shirley, at fifty-three, was feeling enormously fatigued and out of breath, even before she got the flu. She went to her doctor, and while being examined she complained of recurrent chest pain. She said she felt a tug every time she did some minimal activity such as vacuuming or swinging a golf club. Her doctor asked if it was really painful or just annoying, and she answered that she had been handling it pretty well over the years. She was ashamed to make a fuss and wanted to put up a good front for her doctor.

Will Shirley be given an electrocardiogram or thallium stress test? A perceptive doctor would question her closely about her symptoms and medical history. This physician would treat her flu but would *also* investigate her possible long-term heart condition. And a patient who is aware of the possibilities of her symptoms would pursue the correct treatment until she found it.

All too often, this doesn't happen. Recurring angina (chest

pain caused by insufficient blood supply to the heart) is usually ignored by women and their doctors, and even those physicians who acknowledge the problem treat it less aggressively in women than in men. This may mean that there is blockage in multiple arteries before anything is done diagnostically.

DEATH IS CONSIDERED MORE SERIOUSLY THAN LONG-TERM ILLNESS
Diseases that kill quickly, like men's heart disease, command most of the research money and effort in this country. Diseases that create chronic, long-term health problems before they kill, like women's heart disease, generate very little money for research. Statistics that show men dying at early ages receive more attention than those showing women lingering in bad health for many years.

INADEQUATE DRUG TESTING
Most of the clinical trials for heart medications included only men, so it is difficult to judge whether many FDA-approved drugs and their dosages will be as effective in the female body.

From 1977 to 1993, the FDA banned women from early drug trials. Women were specifically excluded because it was thought that they might be in the earliest stages of pregnancy when they signed up for the trials, and the developing fetus might be damaged by the unknown effects of certain drugs. Although this ban has been lifted, there are still fewer clinical trials performed on women than men.

In the past, half of all the drug-safety experiments excluded women, and even those that did include them were judged incorrectly. Since women have more fat content in their bodies than men, a drug that's absorbed and held in fat lingers longer in the body—this means, logically, that a woman can be given a smaller dosage to get the same effect that a man would get. But since the data on drug testing were often not differentiated by sex, no indication was given that various drugs and their side effects affected women differently from men. As a result, these medications might be ineffective or even damaging to the women taking them.

INADEQUATE TREATMENTS

The accepted techniques of treatment, designed by male surgeons for male hearts, are not always as successful when performed on women. Men are recommended for cardiac catheterization and coronary angiography twice as often as women. If women do get catheterized, they are just as likely to undergo balloon angioplasty and bypass surgery as men—however, if their symptoms are ignored, they may never be recommended for these more aggressive procedures. Men are generally operated on at an earlier age, when their outcome might be better than that of an older woman. Twice as many women as men die after bypass surgery, and their rates of success for angioplasty are much lower than men's, for reasons that seem unrelated to age or body size.

INADEQUATE SURGICAL INSTRUMENTATION

Women from ethnic groups and foreign countries who are naturally smaller than Americans of Northern European descent are at even more of a disadvantage. All of the instruments developed for heart surgery were intended for larger male hearts. One of the reasons that the outcome of bypass surgery has been significantly worse for women is that their arteries are smaller and not suited to the equipment used for the procedure. A health-care professional recently reported that her mother, a Cuban-American who weighed under a hundred pounds and was four foot seven, was evaluated for bypass surgery. The decision of the health-care team was that she would have to be moved to the nearest children's hospital. For the operation her surgeon used pediatric equipment with which he was not familiar and which had never been intended to perform this particular type of adult surgery.

Why Are Women Underdiagnosed and Undertreated?

The medical establishment is not entirely to blame for our lack of knowledge and concern about our heart health. First, women are simply not aware that coronary heart disease is a significant problem, one to which they must pay attention. College-educated women tend to know the risks better than those who've only had a high school education or less, but even women with some college background don't know how to protect themselves from the threat of heart disease. Even when symptoms occur, a woman may still remain in the dark about her condition. Very often, a woman who's having chest pain during some activity will stop doing the activity, and sure enough, the chest pain will go away. Is this angina? Or are there other physiological reasons for her muscle spasms? Only accurate tests will say for sure.

Women tend to have fewer routine physicals than men because they generally opt for a visit to the gynecologist once a year instead of a trip to the general practitioner. And even a family doctor may not be attuned to the particular symptoms that would tell a specialist that this woman is a candidate for a heart attack. He may not order the more sensitive cholesterol and triglyceride tests that would give him the information he needs about her lipid levels—her HDLs (high-density lipoproteins, the "good" cholesterol that keeps fat off the arterial walls) and LDLs (low-density lipoproteins, the "bad" cholesterol that allows plaque to collect on the arteries).

Even when diagnosed as having heart disease, women are not treated as aggressively as men. They are more likely to refuse invasive procedures and more willing to use prescription drugs to avoid surgery. These medications can keep a person with heart disease in relatively good health only so long. Will the doctor even consider coronary angioplasty or bypass surgery for a woman? Knowing that the procedures are riskier in a female, he or she may not even suggest it.

Physicians are quick to recommend surgery for men with heart disease—even for those men who might be successfully treated with medicine. So the reason that male surgical survival rates are higher could be that men are operated on even when they aren't sick enough for surgery; whereas women are treated surgically only after medical therapy fails.

And does it make a difference whether our patient sees a male or female physician? *The New England Journal of Medicine* reported in 1993 that women who visited female physicians were more likely to have Pap smears and mammograms. Although there is no clear-cut documentation on whether female physicians more routinely schedule cardiovascular screenings, it is likely that they are more attentive to diseases that might affect their female patients and more persuasive about recommending procedures and preventive tactics that reflect their patients' particular health status.

The numbers now speak for themselves. As do the patients.

"I'd had angina for years, but I never thought I was sick enough to go to the hospital," said Janice, at seventy-one, a healthy woman two years after her heart attack. "So I lay in bed for three days feeling so completely miserable that I couldn't get up and cook for my two sons and their families who'd come to visit. They got so mad at me they finally dragged me to the hospital. It turned out I'd seriously damaged the whole bottom of my heart by waiting so long. And I'm a small woman, so I was a bad candidate for bypass. Did I learn how to exercise and eat right and take my medications after that!"

Sally was only forty-two when her husband threw out his back, so she started doing all the chores around the house. "I thought I had just strained myself when I got this crushing pain in the middle of my chest. It went all the way up to my jaw and down my left arm. I had three blocked arteries, but they could only bypass two because the third was less than a centimeter in size—when they're too small they collapse. I wish I'd known years ago that my mother having a heart attack at thirty-six meant that I was a candidate for early heart disease, too."

Look at the Bigger Picture: A Holistic View of Life

We know that there are certain physical, emotional, and mental risk factors, which will be discussed in detail in Chapter 3. Some clear indicators will help to predict whether you might be a high-risk candidate for heart disease. But there are so many combinations of factors and so many unusual possibilities that no one can tell you for sure where you stand.

This is why it's imperative for you to look at your life—not just the details, but *the whole fiber of your life*—and ask yourself questions that a doctor might never come up with in a case history. In many complementary medical traditions, like homeopathy, and in traditions of other cultures, such as Chinese and Japanese medicine, an accurate diagnosis may depend on such factors as whether you are quick or slow to anger, whether you prefer summer or winter, and whether you are a through-the-night sleeper or take catnaps. All these elements are crucial in the holistic picture that will shift you toward or away from heart disease.

First, you must know the medical parameters:

1. What's your family history?
2. What are your cholesterol, triglyceride, and blood glucose levels?
3. Do you exercise regularly?
4. Are you hypertensive?
5. Are you diabetic?
6. Are you a smoker?
7. Are you postmenopausal, or have you had your ovaries removed (surgical menopause), and if so, do you take replacement estrogen?
8. Do you eat a high-fat, high-cholesterol diet?
9. Are you overweight?

Once you've ascertained your clinical situation, you have to look at the bigger picture. Ask yourself the following and answer honestly:

1. Do you like your life?
2. What are your strengths as an individual?
3. What are your weaknesses?
4. Do you feel comfortable in your body?
5. Do you live in a healthful environment? Are you aware of possible health risks in your house and community?
6. Do you consider yourself a healthy person, or do you have many physical complaints?
7. (If applicable) Are you comfortable living with the family or companions who currently share your life?
8. (If applicable) Are you comfortable living alone?
9. List five major stresses in your life. How do you handle these stresses?
10. When you are upset, are you more typically depressed and sad, or angry?
11. Do you take your anger out on others, or on yourself?
12. Do you make time each day for some period of relaxation or pampering?
13. Do you laugh every day?
14. Do you enjoy—or do you avoid—touching and being touched?
15. Do you allow yourself to cry when it is appropriate to feel sad?
16. Do you believe that you can overcome most difficulties?
17. Are you overwhelmed by most difficulties?
18. How would you change your life, if you could?
19. Do you have a belief system, either spiritual or religious, that carries you through most adversity?
20. Where do you see yourself thirty years from now?

After you've taken this quiz, put it aside for six months as you work through some of the suggestions we'll offer throughout this book. See how your big picture alters as you become aware of what you have to do to maintain a healthy heart.

If You're Healthy Now, You Still Need This Book

If you're only forty now, and you've never had a twinge or a pang, why should you start thinking about your heart? Because heart disease in women is a slow grower, and there's plenty of time left to help or heal ourselves.

We are all living longer. The diseases and conditions that used to take women in their prime have been vanquished—we no longer have to worry about dying in childbirth or succumbing to rheumatic fever. Although tuberculosis has been on the rebound in tightly packed urban areas, most women in this country will never contract TB.

Thanks to better lifelong health habits, high-tech surgical techniques, and improved medications, we can survive to our eightieth birthday and beyond. American women routinely live at least six years longer than most men. We are typically widowed for eleven and a half years of our lives, which means a long time living alone, or with relatives or friends.

Since heart disease in women very often disables rather than kills, the future of America may be significantly altered by those of us who will succumb to coronary conditions. The number of individuals in our society living to eighty-five and beyond has increased enormously—and the generation of baby boomers has produced even more women who will make up a significant proportion of the elderly population of the twenty-first century. Many thousands of women, disabled by heart disease, would strain the resources of federally funded programs like Medicare and Medicaid.

This gloomy scenario is not inevitable. Being eighty-five or ninety years old doesn't have to mean being sick or disabled, in a walker or wheelchair, with a deteriorating body and without mental faculties. Certainly not! Midlife is the time to decide *how* we want to be old. If we cultivate our interests, care for the physical houses in which our souls abide, if we really listen hard to our bodies when they ask for better nutrition and a more appropriate exercise regime, if we settle down and stop reacting to every stressful event as though it is doomsday, we can move effortlessly from midlife to *highlife*.

2

How a Woman's Heart Works

∇

From the earliest years of scientific investigation, people have been pondering just how the heart and circulatory system work. Galen, who was physician to the Roman court in A.D. 130, figured out from his analysis of wounded gladiators that the blood flowed from the body to the heart and then back again to the rest of the body. It took another thousand years for physicians to understand that the blood had to pass through the lungs before returning to the body. And then finally in 1517, Dr. William Harvey came up with our modern description of the circulatory system. He understood that the heart was a muscle that served as a pump, and that it supplied nourishment to the body as it received oxygen from the lungs.

It's not crucial that we understand this legacy of knowledge about the heart. All we need is some background information that will allow us to comprehend what can go wrong and learn how it can be managed. Like Jennifer, a fifty-four-year-old artist, we want to have enough facts at our command to make informed decisions. Until her heart attack, Jennifer had believed—and so had the doctors she'd consulted—that her shortness of breath was the result of a lung problem.

"I was a swimmer, and suddenly I couldn't swim. It just infuriated me to think that age was getting to me, and I resented using the asthma inhaler the doctor had given me. I tried ignoring the messages my body was sending, but I couldn't. I felt too awful.

"The breathing got worse, and it was so hard for me to swim I finally quit smoking. I was scared I might have emphysema. It never occurred to me, or to the doctor I'd seen, that there might be something wrong with my heart.

"Until I was on the plane coming home from a trip to Greece. Suddenly, I felt like an octopus had grabbed my heart and was squeezing the life out of me. It was *crushing* pain, very intense. And somewhere a light went on inside, and I figured it wasn't my lungs, it was my heart.

"I finally decided to see a cardiologist, and she did a catheterization. What I'd experienced on the plane was in fact a heart attack. The doctor found that one of my arteries had shut down completely. But on either side of the damaged artery, two new smaller arteries (my doctor told me they're called collaterals) had been created that fed my other coronary arteries. It was like my heart had made its own bypass! The doctor thought it was all those years of swimming that produced the extra veins.

"I learned a lot about myself from this experience. Since I'm an artist, I'm very selfish about getting what I want when I want it. And because I learned exactly how my heart functions and what it did to save itself, I've developed an enduring faith in my own body. I know it will survive—and so will I."

Jennifer's heart was severely damaged—and yet its own ability to heal itself saved her. Because one area was in trouble, another area compensated and took over the function of the damaged cells.

If we are really to know what went on inside of Jennifer and how her own heart saved her life, we have to look at the whole picture with an anatomist's scrutiny.

How Is the Heart Constructed?

What an inspiring and amazing organ is the human heart! This hollow, muscular pump, an elaborate mechanism that keeps blood moving throughout the body, starts beating about twenty days after conception and keeps going for seventy or eighty—even for one hundred years. It is the core of the circulation system, bringing oxygen and coordinating blood flow to and from the farthest reaches of your body and back again.

We take the amazing resources of the heart for granted, and yet we could not survive without its continuous rhythm, powerful pressure, and its instantaneous adaptations to stress and exercise that go on day and night throughout our entire lifetime.

Where the Heart Lies

The heart sits right in the middle of your chest, protected by the sternum, or breastbone. The apex of the heart points to the left, where the beat is felt. This is why everyone thinks of the heart as located on the left side. About the size of a fist, weighing less than a pound, the pump is a very powerful muscle that responds involuntarily. We don't have to do anything consciously to keep it beating.

The heart is protected by several layers of tissue. On the outside is the **pericardium,** a fibrous sac that shields the heart from surrounding structures (for example, it makes sure that an infection in the lung won't spread to the heart). Inside this sac is the **epicardium,** a membrane that forms the outermost layer of the wall of the heart. Inside the epicardium is the **myocardium,** the middle layer of the heart wall, composed of cardiac muscle. And the inmost layer is the **endocardium,** a very thin smooth layer of cells that lines the inner surface of the heart.

The body contains sixteen pints of blood, and each day, the pump recycles these pints over a thousand times. During an average lifetime, the heart pumps 1.8 million barrels of blood through the body.

The Heart Is Made of Two Pumps and Four Valves

The heart is divided in half by the septum, and each of the two halves is divided into two chambers. On top are the chambers that receive blood—these are the right and left **atria,** which have thin walls; and on the bottom are the chambers that pump blood—the **ventricles,** which have thicker, muscular walls. The left ventricle, which is responsible for pumping blood out to the rest of the body, is the strongest and thickest part of the heart. This is the process of blood flow:

- The right atrium receives the blood that comes from all parts of the body through the veins. This blood is bluish in color because it has exchanged its oxygen for carbon dioxide.
- The right ventricle pumps this venous blood into the lungs, where it is infused with oxygen.
- The left atrium receives oxygenated blood, now deeply red, from the lungs.
- The left ventricle pumps oxygenated blood through the arteries to all the various body tissues.

The rhythm of the heart, well known as the "lub-dub" sound, is caused by the opening and closing of the four **valves** that regulate the flow of blood through the two pumps of the heart.

On the right are the **tricuspid valve** and **pulmonic valve.**

On the left are the **mitral valve** and **aortic valve.**

The valves open to allow blood into a chamber, and as the chamber starts to contract, the valve shuts down so that blood can't flow backward in what's known as a retrograde flow.

As the mitral and tricuspid valves close, we hear the "lub," and as the pulmonic and aortic valves close, we hear the "dub." Other sounds can be caused by improper functioning of the valves. If one of the valves doesn't close completely and some blood flows back, a **murmur** will occur. This can also happen if the valve opening is narrowed. A variety of other sounds may be heard if there's any abnormality or congenital defect of the heart.

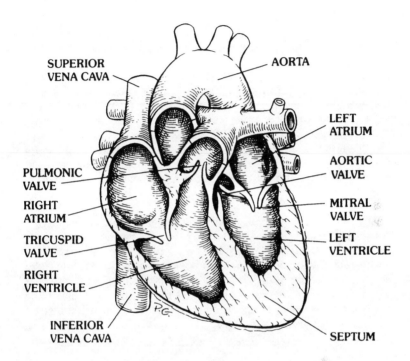

SUPERIOR VENA CAVA

AORTA

LEFT ATRIUM

AORTIC VALVE

PULMONIC VALVE

RIGHT ATRIUM

MITRAL VALVE

TRICUSPID VALVE

LEFT VENTRICLE

RIGHT VENTRICLE

INFERIOR VENA CAVA

SEPTUM

THE HEART AND ITS VALVES

The Electrical System: What Makes the Heart Contract and Beat?

The **sinus node** is the pacemaker for the heart and causes the electrical impulses that generate a beat. Other specialized areas in the heart assist in the function of this conduction system.

The sinus node generates the electric impulse that starts your heartbeat, so this is known as a **sinus rhythm.** The wave coming off this initial impulse travels to every muscle in the atrium, making it contract. The electrical impulse stimulates the other

═══════════════════════════════ ▽ ═══════════════════════════════

What Can Happen If the Heart or Valves Have a Congenital Defect?

A problem can occur if the heart isn't built like the standard-issue pump described above. Women are more prone to being born with defects in the anatomy of the heart. Some of these congenital problems are: **septal defects,** or a hole in the wall that separates two of the chambers of the heart; **congenital aortic stenosis,** where the aortic valve develops less than the three leaflets it should have; **congenital pulmonary stenosis,** a narrowing of the pulmonary valve; **coarctation of the aorta,** where the artery that carries blood from the heart to the body is constricted; and **mitral atresia,** a congenital closure of the mitral valve opening.

Any one of the four valves can develop problems, either through congenital defects, coronary heart disease, or the aging process in general. A valve may develop **stenosis,** where it becomes narrowed and its leaflets don't open and shut properly. A valve can become **leaky** and permit blood to flow in the wrong direction—this is most typical of the mitral valve, where **mitral regurgitation** is a common problem. Any valvular disorder puts a burden on the heart, which compensates by becoming enlarged and weakened.

═══

points of the conduction system, which allows time for the atria to contract and the ventricles to fill.

The electrical impulses of the heart can be charted on an **electrocardiograph** or **ECG.** The tracings that are recorded on graph paper reflect the timing of the beat, the function of the heart muscle itself, and the differences in anatomy that may occur.

What Is Blood Pressure?

The right side of the heart is a low-pressure pump, simply allowing flow into the lungs so that the exchange of carbon

▽
What Could Go Wrong in the Electrical System?

Although there are designated areas that are responsible for establishing and maintaining the beat of the heart, other areas in the atria and ventricles also have the capacity to generate an electrical impulse. If one of these impulses interrupts the ordinary rhythm of the heartbeat, this can set off an irregular heartbeat—an **arrhythmia.** If the normal rhythm is disrupted for a prolonged time, **fibrillation** can result. Atrial fibrillation is benign, however, ventricular fibrillation can result in fainting or death.

dioxide to oxygen can occur. The left side is a high-pressure pump, forcefully ejecting fluid out into the body. **Systolic** blood pressure is determined by the resistance in the arterial wall to the force of blood moving against it. **Diastolic** is the "resting" pressure.

Now what is your physician listening to when she places the **sphygmomanometer,** or blood pressure cuff, on your upper arm?

For each beat of the heart, all chambers must work in perfect harmony and blood must continuously fill each side of the heart. When the thin-walled atria contract, blood is squeezed through the chambers, and then, within seconds, the thick-walled ventricles contract. As the ventricles empty their blood supply, the atria fill with blood again.

The standard healthy blood pressure for a premenopausal woman, set by the National Institutes of Health, should be no more than 140/90. The top figure is measured when the heart contracts and pushes blood into the artery; the bottom figure is the pressure in the arteries when the heart muscle relaxes in between beats. A new heartbeat starts with another contraction in the atria, and so on in an unending **cardiac cycle.**

▽

What Can Go Wrong with Blood Pressure?

When blood pressure is elevated, the heart is forced to work harder in each contraction and relaxes under higher pressure in between beats. By working harder, it increases the force of the blood pushed against the arterial walls, which can damage them. Blood pressure is regulated by a fluid and nerve axis that exists between the kidneys, brain, and blood vessels. If this axis is disrupted, it can elevate blood pressure and vascular tone. Someone with **systemic hypertension** may have thickened and enlarged heart walls. Heart failure can result. The kidneys and the eyes can also be damaged by hypertension.

How Does the Blood Circulate?

The heart could not do its job of nourishing and oxygenating all the cells by itself, and so the body contains a network of miles of blood vessels to carry the blood as it is pumped. Healthy blood vessels are elastic tubes that can stretch, contract, and expand to allow for different blood volumes and pressures.

There are three main types of blood vessels: **arteries** and smaller arteries called **arterioles,** as well as **veins** and **capillaries.** Just like a great river with a network of tributaries, the arteries are largest near the heart and branch out into arterioles, which link up with tiny capillaries that connect to the smallest veins. In turn, one vein feeds into another increasingly larger vein until the blood pours back into the heart, and then goes to the lungs where it can be reoxygenated and start its journey all over again. It is estimated that the blood makes this beautifully charted circuit 2.5 billion times over the course of seventy years of life.

Capillaries. These tiny blood vessels are the filters of the blood system—they are so delicate that food, oxygen, waste products, and carbon dioxide can pass easily across their cell membranes. They connect up with the arteries, which bring food and oxygen to the cells and also with the veins, which carry waste and carbon monoxide away from the cells.

Coronary Arteries. The heart is so busy pumping blood to the rest of the body, it needs its own vascular system to supply it with the blood it needs in order to work. This is the function of the vital coronary arteries, which overlay the heart like a thorny crown. At the top of the heart, these arteries are about as wide as a knitting needle, but they taper down and become thinner as they extend along the outside surface of the heart.

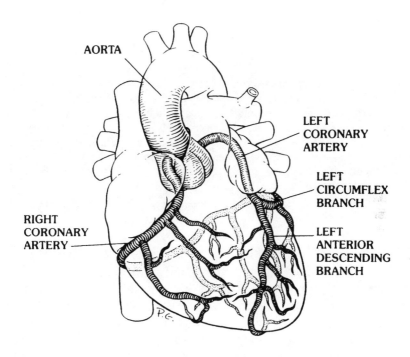

AORTA

LEFT CORONARY ARTERY

LEFT CIRCUMFLEX BRANCH

RIGHT CORONARY ARTERY

LEFT ANTERIOR DESCENDING BRANCH

THE CORONARY ARTERIES

The three coronary arteries—the right, the left circumflex, and the left anterior descending coronary artery—serve to supply the heart muscle with oxygen-rich blood. The right artery nourishes the back of the heart (the inferior wall of the left ventricle), the left anterior descending nourishes the front side and septum, and the left circumflex curves around to nourish the side of the heart. These major arteries connect up with smaller ones along the heart's surface.

What Could Go Wrong with the Coronary Arteries?

Over a period of years, fatty deposits known as plaques can develop on the inside walls of these essential arteries, causing them to narrow in the process known as **atherosclerosis.** As the arteries become increasingly less elastic, it becomes harder for oxygenated blood to flow through the arteries, and slowly the supply may be cut off to the heart and other organs. If a piece of plaque ruptures, a blood clot **(occlusion),** can form and completely block the artery, causing **myocardial infarction,** or a heart attack. In rare cases, an attack may also be caused by a **vascular spasm.**

Veins. These blood vessels run back toward the heart, carrying oxygen-depleted blood. Superficial veins run just under the surface of your skin; deep veins run through the muscles and carry 90 percent of the blood back to your heart; communicating veins carry the blood from superficial to deep veins. Veins have valves, somewhat like the heart, which open upward. This allows blood to move up the vein.

When a muscle contracts, the valve opens and blood is squeezed up the vein. When a muscle relaxes, the valve closes, holding the blood in place.

▽

What Can Go Wrong with the Veins?

Congestive heart failure occurs when the left ventricle cannot pump the amount of blood the body needs. Pressure then mounts in the pulmonary veins, and fluid collects in the lungs and legs, causing shortness of breath and fluid retention, which causes the body to swell. As the heart tries to accommodate the increased pressure on the lungs, the left ventricle cavity dilates and the muscle is "stretched," thus enlarging the heart.

The Biological Differences Between Women and Men

Now that you have a general understanding of the intricate mechanisms that make the heart and circulatory system function, it's time to examine the subtler variations of gender. What you've just learned about the heart is true for both men and women, but there are important differences that make the female heart unique.

First, women are smaller. We have smaller skeletons, smaller internal organs, and smaller hearts. The female heart weighs about 50 to 100 grams less than a man's, and it beats more often and more quickly both at rest and in motion to meet the body's needs. The more we work our heart by stressing it well with exercise, the more effective the heart muscle becomes.

Not only is a woman's heart smaller, her coronary arteries (and in fact all her arteries and veins) are also typically smaller. This means that it takes less plaque to occlude a woman's artery than it would a man's.

If a woman does require surgery on these arteries, the question always arises as to whether her vessels will accommodate standard surgical instruments. Janice, whom we met in the last chapter, had three occluded arteries, but only two were acceptable for bypass. At seventy-one, Janice was not in poor physical condition, but she weighed only 108 pounds and stood five feet tall. Her third artery was less than a centimeter in size, and therefore inoperable. There isn't much room inside a very small blood vessel, and when the passageway is too narrow to begin with, there's a greater chance that it will close up again shortly after a balloon procedure or surgery.

In addition to producing estrogen, women may be protected in their early years from heart disease by their higher insulin production. Insulin, which regulates the way that glucose (blood sugar) is supplied to the body, has a beneficial effect on the HDL cholesterol. It also works to open the blood vessels and allows blood to flow through more easily, reducing the force of the blood pressure. One major reason that diabetes is a risk factor for heart disease is because it inhibits the body from creating and using insulin effectively.

Although the standard exercise treadmill test is a good barometer of the way a man's heart responds to stress, it's not the same for women. The reason this type of test is an uncertain procedure for women is that the female heart, when enduring exercise, may produce ECG patterns that can be interpreted as abnormal although they're not. For this reason, many physicians will only credit a treadmill test if it is accompanied by an echocardiogram or is done with a radionuclide dye such as thallium or Cardiolite. (See Chapter 8 on testing.)

Women's hearts react differently from men's hearts to physical and emotional stress, and this has great bearing on the function of our hearts. The stress response is regulated by the **autonomic** or **involuntary nervous system,** which also controls the heartbeat. When we are in a fearful or difficult situation, the part of our brain that signals "danger" triggers a release of certain neurochemicals that allow us to act quickly. This "fight or flight" response triggers a rush of adrenaline through our system. When this happens, our blood pressure rises, our heart speeds up, our stomach clenches, and our pupils dilate. Irregular heartbeats (arrhythmias) can result from a stress reaction to terror.

Grace, whom we will meet in a later chapter, was misdiagnosed in the emergency room three times. She said that she became more hysterical each time as the doctors tried to tell her she had an ulcer, when she knew deep down that she had had a heart attack. Her agitation and fury at the incompetence of the medical professionals around her brought up a rush of stress hormones, which may have exacerbated her already serious condition and may have contributed to the severity of her heart attack.

Although men and women both experience this stress response, it is interesting to see how they differ in what happens next. Men often perceive stress as a good thing (eu-stress), a challenge to their abilities and an opportunity to triumph over duress. Many physicians credit the ability of type A men to bounce back after a heart attack to their determination to get back to the pressure of their jobs as quickly as possible. They may produce the same stress hormones, but they will stop producing them as soon as they vent their anger and "take care" of the problem at hand.

Women, however, who may have been conditioned from childhood to choke back their anger or repress their emotions, often see stress as a major obstacle (dis-stress) and allow it to overwhelm them. Their "fight or flight" response is continuous, keeping the stress hormone level unnaturally high all the time. If we permit enough stress to invade our days and weeks, we are inviting more disruption of our normal heart pattern.

How Women Change Hormonally Across the Life Span

Because of our biological heritage, we have several life experiences unknown to men. In our first or growth stage of life, we go through puberty and begin to menstruate; during our second or reproductive stage, we are able to conceive and bear children, and we can lactate and nourish new life; and as we enter the third stage of maturation, we go through menopause as our menstrual cycle stops. These significant events make a huge difference in the health of the female heart.

The reason is the gonadal hormone **estrogen,** which men also produce but in much smaller quantities. (Men's counterpart hormone is testosterone, which women also make and utilize, although to a far lesser extent.) Estrogen is the leading player in female heart health up to menopause, when menses stops and the gonadal hormonal output drops to within 20 percent of its former peak in the reproductive years.

Estrogen plays several crucial roles in our early life that generally afford us cardiovascular protection that men don't have. Although some women have heart attacks in their twenties and thirties, these individuals tend to have unusually strong family histories of heart disease that override their hormonal protection. For most women, estrogen is one of the best defenses against heart disease because:

• Estrogen is a primary influence on the way that the body handles lipids—the fats we produce and ingest. Since heart disease and heart attacks are often caused by the deposition of fats inside the arteries, estrogen is our trump card in the early years of our campaign for a healthy heart. About a third to a half of estrogen's protective effect has to do with maintaining a good balance between high-density and low-density lipoproteins (HDLs and LDLs).

• Estrogen has a direct effect on the coronary arteries, which contain estrogen receptors. The hormone inhibits or retards plaque formation by blocking the incorporation of low-density lipoproteins—the "bad" cholesterol—into the artery walls. During our reproductive years, we have the advantage over men because estrogen keeps our high-density lipoproteins (HDLs) high, and our low-density lipoproteins (LDLs) relatively low. But when we lose estrogen later in life, the balance shifts, and we have no more protection than men do against heart disease.

• Estrogen helps to maintain the vascular tone of blood vessel walls, keeping them elastic and flexible.

How Our Estrogen Affects Us Through the Stages of Life

Let's look at the way estrogen affects our health as we grow from childhood to womanhood:

Childhood to Puberty. In the beginning, boys and girls have an equal balance of fats, or lipids, in their bloodstreams. The HDLs and LDLs of normal children are similar, regardless of sex. But between the ages of ten and twelve, as we enter puberty, we gain an advantage over boys. The rapid boost in their testosterone production causes their HDLs to fall, while the boost we get from the start-up of estrogen causes our HDLs to rise.

Adolescence. During adolescence, hormonal fluctuation is the norm, and the sex hormone levels rise and fall dramatically, sometimes daily. You will undoubtedly remember the unpredictability of periods, the skin eruptions, and the moodiness that seemed to take over your emotional and physical life. This erratic seesaw may have lasted until age eighteen or twenty, when your hormonal patterns settled into a calm rhythm.

Reproductive Years. The cycle is now established, as is the hormonal ebb and flow. During the first twelve days of your cycle, estrogen is the predominant hormone, keeping HDLs high and reducing LDLs. Remember, too, that estrogen is a mood elevator, so you're more likely to feel positive and upbeat during the first half of your cycle.

At ovulation, when an egg is released from the ovary for its trip down the fallopian tubes and into the uterus, estrogen levels fall for a few days and progesterone, the hormone that acts as a counterbalance to the system, begins to proliferate. About seven days after ovulation, estrogen rises again and comes back up to reach a second peak.

But during the second half of the cycle, progesterone is the predominant hormone. It does have a depressing effect on mood (this is the time when PMS symptoms may appear), but at this time of your life, it does not elevate LDLs.

If the egg is not fertilized, the levels of both estrogen and progesterone fall steadily until the end of the cycle. HDLs and

LDLs are not adversely affected by these fluctuations during the reproductive years.

Pregnancy. Let's see what happens to the heart if the egg is fertilized. Estrogen and progesterone levels are the highest they have ever been as they work to keep up the ever-changing bed for the implanted egg that is growing daily. All lipid levels rise early in pregnancy, but HDLs drop at about twenty-four weeks of gestation. This isn't something to be terribly concerned about, since a pregnant woman still has an HDL level that is about 15 percent higher than a nonpregnant woman. LDLs stay high until well after delivery.

The rise in hormonal levels is also responsible for a tendency to retain water and salt, which help your body gain weight during the pregnancy. By the fifth month, your blood volume will have increased by almost half. When your body has that much more blood to pump, your heart must work harder—it beats ten to twenty times more per minute. All of this blood requires more oxygen, so the more you exercise during pregnancy, the more you breathe and the more oxygen you provide your blood and your heart.

Blood pressure usually falls during pregnancy, but it is still important for you to keep it under control with diet and exercise. If you are hypertensive to begin with, your physician will monitor you closely so that the increased burden of pregnancy won't endanger you.

During labor, the heart has to work 30 percent harder than usual, and by the time you're delivering your baby, your heart may be working four or five times more than it did in its nonpregnant state.

If you were diagnosed with heart disease before becoming pregnant, you will be tested regularly to make sure that you and your baby are safe and that your heart is performing as it should.

Midlife. As we mature, our first estrogen peak prior to ovulation gets higher and the second peak doesn't rise as high. (This is one reason why it becomes increasingly difficult to get pregnant and stay pregnant in your forties.) As we approach menopause, LDL levels rise significantly and HDLs drop a little. The body is not as finely balanced as it was in earlier years. Finally, we run out of viable eggs in our ovaries, and the brain receives the message that ovulation is no longer occurring. When this occurs, a woman goes through menopause and no longer ovulates or menstruates.

Postmenopause. Although a woman still produces some estrogen in her adrenal glands, she usually doesn't have enough to keep her arteries in the best shape. Her HDLs fall, but the really big change is that her LDLs rise sharply, allowing plaque to accumulate on coronary arteries. This dramatically increases her risk of heart disease.

Women in previous generations didn't often live past menopause, so the problem of keeping a healthy heart until advanced old age simply never came up. But today, with a woman's life expectancy in America at seventy-eight or even higher, it is clearly imperative that she consider what the loss of estrogen does to the quality and quantity of her later years. In Chapter 6 you can learn about the possibility of medically replacing the estrogen and progesterone you lose with age.

This is not to say that estrogen is the entire story when it comes to heart health. As we will see in later chapters, there are women who have heart attacks below the age of forty, when the hormones are at peak levels. But many other factors (see Chapter 3) could cause such an early cardiac event in an otherwise healthy individual.

Pay Attention to the Body

When you know something about the way the heart works and how physiological changes across the life span can affect it, you are better prepared to understand what your cardiovascular liabilities and assets really are. We are all built so differently, and yet, since the master plan is the same, we have good parameters for determining just how much risk we have.

In the next chapter, you will be able to look at all your personal risks—some of which you undoubtedly never knew might make you more susceptible to heart disease. Looking at the whole picture will open your eyes to new possibilities. You can fine-tune your heart health by changing certain elements, if you have to, and monitoring others.

You are more than just a collection of blood vessels and valves, and you have the potential to improve your well-being as you begin to make use of all facets—physical, mental, emotional, social—that can help you to become a healthier woman over the years.

3

What Are Your Risk Factors for Heart Disease?

▽

It is absolutely vital that every woman know exactly what her risk is for heart disease. It has been clearly shown that preventive care makes a difference—if you change certain elements in your life, you can avoid heart attacks or chronic heart disease.

If you are a smoker with high blood pressure and high cholesterol, if you are an overweight, postmenopausal couch potato, you are at high risk for heart disease. But there's a lot you can do—even if you have multiple risk factors—to change your situation. When you understand the dangers inherent in your lifestyle, you can do something about them.

Katharine, who at fifty-two is childless and unmarried, has undergone not only a heart attack but also triple bypass surgery. She used to be a housekeeper, but she's been disabled for the last eight years because of her heart condition and the ruptured disk in her back. Katharine is still overweight, but she has her diabetes and hypertension under control and exercises several times a week at the program run in her apartment complex. After years of trying to ignore her condition, she now knows her risks and is finally beginning to reduce them.

"When I look back and see what I did to myself, it's hard to figure. I smoked all my life, and I ate whatever I wanted. So that night at the bingo game, when I felt the terrible pain from the back of my chest going to the front, I guess I shouldn't have been too surprised. My sister called an ambulance in time, thank God.

"The next morning, there I was in intensive care with all these tubes and wires sticking out of me. I wasn't scared; I just thanked God I was alive. I'd always thought that when you have a heart attack, you die.

"Even after my heart attack—and that was eight years ago—and even knowing that I had multiple risks, I just couldn't get myself to do what the doctor said. I'd go along with the program for a while, and I'd feel okay, so I'd light up again. Then I had to have the bypass, and it was still hard for me to stop. But last September I watched my brother die of lung cancer, and I went home and threw my last pack out. That was it. I stayed on my Captopril for the hypertension, and I take a diuretic too. I saw the nutritionist for my diabetes and the heart condition, and I went back to exercising.

"The thing is, I have to take even more care, because my whole family had heart problems. I lost my mother before my heart attack, then my sister, with whom I'd lived for thirty years, died in her sleep. My two brothers went within a year of each other. It's important for me to take care of myself now, because there's no one to take care of me. I have to pay attention to the way I live, maybe more than other people do."

Katharine had a great number of risk factors that might have precipitated her heart attack. She was overweight, hypertensive, diabetic, postmenopausal, and African-American. Even after her heart attack, she wasn't able to make enough changes to protect her in the years that followed. And now she suffers from a lot of stress—she can't work because she's disabled, and over the past seven years, she lost most of her family, the people closest to her. She is struggling to change her lifestyle, and what she's done is significant. But she knows she can do more—and that's the key. She won't stop trying, for the sake of her heart.

Who's at Risk for Heart Disease?

There are very few individuals in the civilized world today whose hearts are not in jeopardy. Thanks to the comforts of modern civilization, most of us have succumbed to the perils of luxury—we all move around too little, worry more than we should, and eat too much of foods that are detrimental to our health. In autopsies done on children under the age of three, it was evident that plaque had already begun to develop on their tiny arteries. If we put ourselves in such jeopardy so early in life, how much damage has been done by the time we are forty, fifty, or sixty years old? And is there any way to predict whether the risks we run will necessarily doom us to a life of chronic illness? Or can we turn the tables and reverse our predisposition for heart disease?

How do you know what your risk is? If you are a perfectly healthy thirty-year-old woman who eats a balanced diet, goes to a health club once a week, and stopped smoking five years ago, should you be concerned? It is hard to say at this point. It may make a great difference how you treat yourself and what happens in the next twenty or thirty years.

Now, if you are a sixty-year-old woman who walks two miles a day and religiously avoids fat in your diet, but your father died of a heart attack, should you be concerned? Probably. The fact that you are postmenopausal increases your risk considerably, even if you're a health nut. But your family history is an even more persuasive factor. On the other hand, if you are aware of your heart health status and take some giant steps to reduce other risks, you may be able to alter your genetic destiny.

When you look at heart disease from a holistic perspective, you will understand that many factors—some physical, some psychological, some social—make you more or less susceptible to getting ill. Although you are handed certain factors you cannot change, you can make enough of a difference in the factors that are under your control to alter radically your chances of staying well. The more risk factors you have, the greater your likelihood of developing heart disease. The more risk factors you moderate or eliminate, the better your likelihood of good health.

You are born a woman, so unless you have a strong family history of heart disease, you are protected by your hormones during your reproductive years. You lose that protection as you age and your stores of estrogen decrease. But if you choose to take hormone replacement therapy, it is conceivable that you can alter this risk.

You are aging daily, and once you have reached those critical years when hormonal balance works against your heart, you are in a danger zone. However, if you change your lifestyle sufficiently, working with all the factors in the second risk category—diet, exercise, attitude, and stress reduction—you may effectively make your biological age younger than your chronological age and beat your own odds on heart disease.

Nothing is carved in stone. You are ultimately in charge of nearly every facet of your heart profile.

Because you need your own personalized guide for self-evaluation, we're going to separate all the various elements for you. Understand, however, that the parts are not always a good picture of the whole. The person you are, your approach to work and play, and your various lifestyle choices and priorities will all weigh heavily in whether or not you develop heart disease. If your cholesterol is high, you can lower it—either with diet and exercise or with medication or both. That's not such a difficult chore for most individuals. But if you deal poorly with stress and your attitude toward aging and illness is negative and fearful, you will have a great deal of work to do.

Take the quiz at the end of this chapter, then put it aside for several months as you work to reduce or eliminate some of your risks. Then take the test again and see how you've improved your heart health status. The good numbers you see will encourage you to do even more to protect yourself from heart disease.

_____▽_____

Risk Factors You Cannot Control

Sex: Being a woman and producing estrogen reduces your risk of heart disease in your reproductive years.

Age: Past fifty or fifty-five, you no longer have the protection of the hormone estrogen, and by sixty-five your risk equals that of a man the same age.

Family History: If you have one or more immediate family members who had heart disease or a heart attack below the age of fifty-five, you are at higher risk yourself.

Race: African-American, Hispanic, and some Native American women tend to have more risk factors than Caucasian women.

Risk Factors You Can Control or Manage

Cholesterol Levels: HDLs should be higher than 45; LDLs lower than 130; total less than 200.

Triglycerides: Level should be below 200.

Hypertension: Systolic pressure should be under 140; diastolic pressure should be under 90.

Diabetes: The disease known as diabetes mellitus interferes with the body's ability to balance blood sugar levels and can also lower HDL cholesterol. Some women with diabetes also have higher blood pressure. (Since you may have a genetic predisposition to this disease, it is not always a controllable factor, but it can be managed.)

Weight: You should not be more than 20 percent over desired weight as determined by life insurance tables.

Stress: Feeling pressured and overwhelmed produces hormones that may trigger arrhythmias and raise blood pressure.

Smoking: Nicotine raises blood pressure; toxins damage artery walls. Smoking can also lead to blood clots and constricted blood vessels in legs, kidney, heart, and brain.

Smoking and Birth Control Pills: The dosage of estrogen and progesterone in birth control pills accentuates the body's ability to form clots. This, in combination with smoking cigarettes, can lead to heart attack, stroke, or pulmonary embolism.

Multiple pregnancies: If you have borne five or more children, your HDL levels may be suppressed.

Alcohol: Overconsumption of alcohol can lead to liver damage, mental disorders, accident, and injury. Women do not produce sufficient stomach enzymes to process the toxins in large amounts of alcohol.

Social Status: Poor, uneducated women tend to know less about health care and may not be able to afford the services of medical professionals.

Social Isolation: Women who are isolated have more difficulty taking care of themselves physically and having the emotional impetus to get well and stay well.

Let's examine these elements in more detail.

Risk Factors You Cannot Control

SEX

Being a woman and producing estrogen reduces your risk of heart disease in your reproductive years. This hormone keeps high-density lipoprotein (HDL) levels elevated because it accelerates fat storage and carbohydrate conversion for eventual conception and nourishment of a fetus. Estrogen also helps maintain blood vessel elasticity to accommodate the increased blood volume we develop when we're pregnant.

Although men secrete a small amount of estrogen, their predominant gonadal, or sex, hormone is testosterone. Testosterone amplifies the body's ability to produce muscle mass and carry oxygen—two beneficial aspects that are somewhat mitigated by the way they affect low-density lipoprotein (LDL) production.

LDL levels rise when muscles contract because the membranes around them become depleted and need more cholesterol to build them back up again. If the body is inactive, the LDLs don't produce muscle but instead build up in the blood and clog arteries. Evidently, the more a woman exercises, the better.

AGE

Women's hearts are usually protected until menopause by their abundance of the hormone estrogen. (There are certainly women with strong family histories of heart disease who have heart attacks under the age of forty, because their genetic potential overwhelms their hormonal protection, but this is not common.) But during the period following the cessation of menses (from about forty-nine to fifty-five, for most American women) estrogen levels drop to within 20 percent of their former peak. And during the next ten years, the activity of plaque formation and vasoconstriction (the tendency of blood vessels to narrow) accelerates. This means that at about age sixty-five, a woman's risk of contracting heart disease rises to equal that of a man the same age.

Being older means that it is more dangerous to be ill. By the time a woman seeks a diagnosis about her cardiac condition, she has more symptoms and more damage has been done to her system. Her chances for healing well or even surviving major surgery are not as good as they would be were she younger and healthier. Older people tend to have lowered immunity and less resilience and ability to bounce back from a traumatic event than their younger counterparts. The older we are when we contract heart disease, the greater our chances of having some other complicating disease or dysfunction.

FAMILY HISTORY

If you have a parent, grandparent, or sibling who developed heart disease at an early age (under fifty-five for men, under sixty-five for women), you are at higher risk than those who have no immediate family member with the condition. The more close relatives you have who meet this criterion, the higher your risk. People with two immediate family members with heart disease are five to ten times more likely to develop it themselves.

The condition is not genetic—that is, you have no strand of DNA that determines your getting the disease as you do your eye color. However, you may be predisposed to getting the disease if it is already in your family.

Although family history counts for a lot, and it is *basically* out of your hands, it is not a completely immutable factor. In examining your risk potential in light of family history, you must also know what kind of lifestyle your sick relatives led. If they were all nonexercising smokers who ate a high-fat diet, and you have an exemplary lifestyle, you are probably more than one up on your original odds. But you may have to work harder at diet, exercise, and stress reduction than a person with no family history of heart disease.

RACE

More African-American and Hispanic women and some Native American women have multiple risk factors for heart disease than Caucasian women. Poor women of color are likely to be overweight—partly because of lack of knowledge about nutrition, partly because they may not be able to afford a good diet—and this liability contributes to other risk factors such as hypertension, diabetes, and high cholesterol levels. We don't have a great deal of specific information on the differences in heart abnormalities as they relate to race because so few women of color have been studied and tested. Most of the research on heart disease has used Caucasian men as the barometer.

Not all risk factors affect all racial groups the same way. Even though Native American women have high rates of obesity and diabetes, they have low incidence of heart disease. For some unknown reason, they are able to maintain lower total cholesterol and lower LDLs. According to studies at the Rush Medical College in Chicago and at the National Institutes of Health Laboratory in Phoenix, Arizona, the Pima Indians in the southwestern United States seem to have a group genetic disposition to carrying a form of LDL that's actually protective against heart disease. This particular type of LDL passes off cholesterol onto the HDLs, which in turn are responsible for transporting it out of the body in the urine, feces, and sweat.

Risk Factors You Can Control or Manage

CHOLESTEROL LEVELS

You are at higher risk for heart disease if your total cholesterol level is over 200. But more important than the total number is the balance of your HDLs to LDLs. To keep your arteries in the best shape possible, your HDL should be above 45, your LDL below 130, and your triglycerides (we'll discuss this other type of lipid in a moment) below 200.

HDLs keep plaque off the arteries and have a beneficial effect on the heart. LDLs are smaller and denser and attach easily to blood vessel walls, eventually narrowing them and obstructing blood flow.

You can factor out your cholesterol level with the following formula (as long as you don't have triglycerides over 300):

LDL = total cholesterol − (triglycerides ÷ 5) − HDL.

You can't raise HDLs with diet, only with exercise, estrogen, smoking cessation, and certain medications. But a diet that's low in cholesterol and saturated fat, high in fiber and complex carbohydrates, *will* lower LDLs. Unfortunately, in comparing groups of men and women on a very low fat diet, the benefit to women was less than the benefit to men. LDLs and triglycerides fell less in women than in men.

This was also the case when some other lipid regulators were changed. Increasing exercise and losing weight were both more effective for men, as was controlling diabetes.

There's another interesting sidelight to the effects of cholesterol on a woman's cardiovascular system. A particular type of LDL known as Lp(a) (pronounced "lp little a") has been identified as the most powerful trigger of strokes. Lp(a) is genetically determined and cannot be altered by diet or exercise the way regular LDLs can. A study at Baylor College in Texas showed that taking hormone replacement therapy—estrogen plus a progestin—can reduce Lp(a) by 50 percent. The hormones appear to make the liver more efficient in removing LDL cholesterol. (See Chapter 6 for more information on hormone replacement therapy.)

Although you can't take steps to reduce your risk of stroke from an abundance of Lp(a), you can still lower your general risk by being cautious when it comes to ingesting cholesterol and fats. **Hyperlipidemia**—or elevation of lipid levels—is a serious risk factor for coronary artery disease. Stopping smoking and taking cholesterol-regulating medications (if your doctor prescribes them) will raise your HDLs. But your two best sources of high HDLs are estrogen and, to a certain extent, aerobic exercise.

You can and should alter your diet to eliminate saturated fats and keep your LDLs low. Reading and understanding food labels (see Chapter 4) could be a lifesaver.

TRIGLYCERIDES

The lipid triglyceride can be an independent risk factor for heart disease in women. People who are diabetic, obese, suffer from thyroid dysfunction or abuse alcohol all have elevated triglyceride levels. Cigarette smoking and lack of exercise can also bump levels up. Women naturally have higher triglyceride levels than men, and these levels appear to signal heart disease more than it would in men. The current thinking is that levels should be kept between 50 and 200 mg/dl, depending on a person's age (since levels rise naturally as we grow older).

HYPERTENSION

The persistent elevation of your blood pressure above 140/90 classifies as hypertension, which means, in effect, that your heart is being forced to work against greater resistance than it should.

How does this occur? If you have arteries already clogged with plaque, the passageway for circulation is narrowed, and the heart has to pump harder to get the blood through. This heightened pressure can create "shear stresses" on artery walls, which may disrupt or rupture already existing plaques. When plaques rupture, they can activate the body's clotting system and lead to occlusions, heart attacks, or strokes.

About 10 percent of American adults suffer from "silent" hypertension. They have no particular symptoms and therefore may not consult a physician for this condition until there is damage not only to the heart, but also possibly to the brain and kidneys as well.

Two times as many women of color over the age of twenty-five have hypertension than white women. Postmenopausal females of all races have it more than they did in their reproductive years. More women over sixty-five have high blood pressure than men of the same age. You are at higher risk for hypertension if you are diabetic, obese, a smoker, or a big consumer of caffeine.

Essential hypertension—the most common form—has no particular underlying cause. But about 10 percent of all cases are called **secondary hypertension,** and these stem from some other disorder such as kidney disease, adrenal gland dysfunction, or a congenital problem. Secondary hypertension is more common in women than in men.

Although we think of stress as an elevator of blood pressure, food can do it too. Sodium—salt—is the primary culprit because of the way it affects several different body systems. It elevates the fluid volume in the body, since it keeps the kidneys from excreting fluids properly. It also affects the sympathetic nervous system, making it more reactive to stress hormones. A low-salt diet can reduce blood pressure as much as 10 points systolic and 5 points diastolic, for example, from 140/90 to 130/85. Some individuals are extremely sensitive to sodium, and these people are at highest risk from a diet heavy in salt.

It may sound strange, but some people only have hypertension when they're in the doctor's office. There are some individuals who are so upset and nervous during a medical examination that their blood pressure elevates unnaturally. This is called "white coat" hypertension, because merely the sight of a medical professional's garb can cause it. If you have no other risk factors, you might want to try taking your blood pressure over several readings at different times of day in a public setting (many drugstores now have blood pressure cuffs). Make sure you don't talk when you're having your pressure taken, because even a simple conversation will raise blood pressure.

DIABETES

A diabetic woman has a risk equal to that of a man of having a heart attack—no matter what her age. She doesn't have the gift of the extra ten or fifteen years' grace period most women enjoy. And several recent studies show that diabetic women were more likely than diabetic men to develop heart disease and to die during their hospitalization following a heart attack or within the next year.

Diabetes is a catchall for several different disorders. Its actual meaning is "excessive excretion of urine," but this symptom shows up for different reasons, depending on the type of illness you have.

The most common form of diabetes is **diabetes mellitus,** which hits one woman in ten. And the particular form that appears in women over forty is called **noninsulin dependent** or **Type II diabetes.** This condition is caused by a failure of certain cells in the pancreas to produce enough insulin to allow the tissues to absorb glucose. The heavier the individual—and many diabetics are obese—the more insulin receptors she has. However, the greater number of receptors does not ensure proper use of the insulin produced. When the body doesn't have enough insulin, or can't properly use the insulin it does make, blood sugar levels rise to abnormal levels and the glucose is excreted in the urine.

Type II diabetes is common in overweight women who have a high sugar content in their diets, and it may develop gradually after bouts of chronic pancreatitis or an adverse reaction to oral contraceptives or corticosteroid drugs, which are often prescribed for treatment of arthritis or allergies. Some women who develop gestational diabetes during their pregnancies and give birth to babies who weigh over nine pounds (probably because of their mothers' high blood sugar) may be at risk for diabetes mellitus in later life.

The condition also has a strong genetic component, so if your parents or siblings have diabetes, you are at increased risk of developing it. Your ethnic background is also significant—the condition is more prevalent in Native American, Hispanic, and African-American women. Hypertension also puts you at risk for this disease.

Unfortunately, if you are a woman, no matter your age, diabetes also increases your risk for heart disease fivefold—at least twice the risk of men with diabetes. This condition was found to be a determinant of coronary heart disease, a certain type of stroke, and nonfatal heart attacks, as well as death from cardiovascular disease. Why is this so?

A woman who contracts diabetes in midlife tends to have accumulated additional risks already. She is probably overweight and may be hypertensive. As she loses the protective effects of estrogen on her heart, her lipid profile (how many HDLs and LDLs she has and in what proportion) tends to worsen. Diabetes lowers HDL cholesterol while it increases LDL cholesterol and triglycerides. It also makes a woman more susceptible to developing a blood clot and to damaging the lining of the blood vessels in the heart from high blood sugar and insulin levels. The chance of developing heart disease when you have established diabetes is obviously greater when other risks—smoking, hypertension, high cholesterol, and obesity—are also present. Finally, diabetes creates changes in your nerve fibers and may deaden your sensation of pain. You may suffer a "silent" heart attack and simply not feel it.

And age compounds these factors. The older you are, the more damage diabetes has done to the various systems of your body. This makes it harder for lifestyle alteration, medication, and surgery to effect positive changes that would protect your heart.

If you've been experiencing enormous thirst, fatigue, blurred vision, weight loss, and frequent urination, you should speak to your doctor about having a glucose test. If you find that you do have diabetes and can get it under control, you will also be protecting your heart.

WEIGHT

You are obese, and therefore at higher risk for heart disease, if you are 20 percent or more above the average weight range for your height as determined by the Society of Actuaries and Association of Life Insurance Medical Directors of America. A follow-up to the Framingham Heart Study showed that obese women were twice as likely as women of normal weight to develop coronary artery disease, and that the risk rose as the individual's weight rose. Only age and blood pressure were more significant in predicting whether or not a woman would develop this condition.

As of March 1990, one in five adults—thirty-four million American—fall into this category.

If you are African-American, you are twice as likely as a Caucasian woman to be obese—this often reflects lifestyle, education, and economic status. If you don't have the money to afford a good diet and don't understand how your health is affected by what you eat and how you exercise, you could easily tend to put on pounds.

But *where* you put the pounds is the most important indicator of how weight will affect your heart health. The *gynoid* or "pear-shape" is the healthy one to have, regardless of how you think it looks to be bottom heavy.

The dangerous "apple" or *android* body shape, where the fat is carried in the upper abdomen, perilously close to the heart, can be a predictor of future coronary heart disease in and of itself, no matter what you weigh. Women should have a waist-to-hip ratio of less than 0.8. We all have to be more careful about body shape as we age and our estrogen levels drop because the deposition of our fat tends to change.

An interesting sidelight to this risk factor is that apple-shaped women tend to produce more of the stress hormone cortisol than pear-shaped women. A study at Yale University showed high amounts of cortisol in the saliva of forty-one overweight women with a lot of fat around their stomach and chest area. The curious body/mind connection with this finding was that the apple-shaped women kept their stress and anger under wraps, whereas the pear-shaped women let out their hostility.

The Nurses' Health Study, begun in 1976 on a group of 121,000 nurses from the ages of thirty-five to fifty-five, ended in 1984. During this time, after adjusting for age and smoking, the rate of nonfatal heart attacks and fatal coronary heart disease combined was only 32 per 100,000 in the thinnest women. The rate was an astounding 106 per 100,000 in the heaviest group. The study showed that 70 percent of heart disease occurred in obese women. There are numerous other studies that indicate the severity of risk from being considerably overweight.

WOMEN

Height	Small Frame	Medium Frame	Midpoint Reference	+10%	+20%	Large Frame
4'10"	102–111	109–121	115	127	138	118–131
4'11"	103–113	111–123	117	129	140	120–134
5' 0"	104–115	113–126	120	132	144	122–137
5' 1"	106–118	115–129	122	134	146	125–140
5' 2"	108–121	118–132	125	138	150	128–143
5' 3"	111–124	121–135	128	141	154	131–147
5' 4"	114–127	124–138	131	144	157	134–151
5' 5"	117–130	127–141	134	147	161	137–155
5' 6"	120–133	130–144	137	151	164	140–159
5' 7"	123–136	133–147	140	154	168	143–163
5' 8"	126–139	136–150	143	158	172	146–167
5' 9"	129–142	139–153	146	161	175	149–170
5'10"	132–145	142–156	149	164	179	152–173
5'11"	135–148	145–159	152	167	182	155–176
6' 0"	138–151	148–162	155	170	186	158–179

Height/Weight chart adapted from Metropolitan Life's *Height & Weight Tables for Men and Women.*

You don't have to be as skinny as a model to protect your heart—and it can be disastrous to drop to a weight lower than what your metabolism and build should support. However, if you are considerably over your desired weight range, it is essential that you consider what you are doing to yourself. We'll discuss just what to eat and what kinds of activity to do in the next chapter, but the first step is acknowledging your risk. You cannot deny such a potent force in your heart health.

STRESS

Stress is a risk factor for heart disease because it raises blood pressure and causes us to produce certain neurochemicals—the "fight or flight" response. When we can't handle stress, our hormones surge, and we often feel our heart pounding. Our stress hormones have the facility to keep LDL cholesterol circulating in the bloodstream longer, which can eventually lead to plaque buildup. Increased blood pressure also may break down the lining of the blood vessels of the heart allowing fat droplets to be deposited inside their delicate walls. Thus stress can lead to cell damage, which can lead to atherosclerosis.

Stress is a constant companion of most women. It is not easy to live in the modern world, whether you are single or partnered, a housewife, a working mother or grandmother, or a corporation president. Pressures about relating to your own and the other sex are common, and are reinforced by media images of "happy" family life. You may be stressed about your children's well-being or stressed because you never had children. If you have living elderly parents, you are undoubtedly pressured to be a good daughter, take care of them in their old age, and never complain. If you are a parent of grown children, you may worry more over their financial and familial woes than you do over your own.

Some new research has investigated whether women in the workplace are more at risk for heart disease than women at home. The fascinating findings indicate that women in executive positions, who are in charge and able to make decisions, are not at greater risk. Women in blue-collar jobs who are unable to exert any control over what they do or how they do it and who must also contain their hostility and anger toward unreasonable bosses' demands are certainly at greater risk. This problem is compounded when a woman must juggle a job she hates with a demanding spouse and difficult child-care arrangements. The stress itself, then, is not the issue—but how much you can do to mold it and manage it.

Your living environment also causes stress—phones that ring, cars that won't start, radon in the basement—and your job— whatever it is. You can't get ahead the way you'd like, or you feel that your responsibilities are too great. You try to divide your time between home and office but rarely succeed. And there's even a pressure in our society to have fun!

All these stresses combine and fold back on one another. Although men may have just as many stresses as women, we tend to "take them to heart" more. Which means that women who don't cope well with stress may be causing a lot of emotional and biochemical damage to their hearts with their abundance of stress hormones. Learning to deal well with the stresses we do have is more realistic than getting rid of stress altogether. We'll discuss this in Chapter 5.

SMOKING

Smoking may be the most deadly risk factor presented in this chapter. Women smokers are two to six times as likely as nonsmokers of having a heart attack and are 60 percent more likely to have coronary artery disease.

Smoking damages the body in a variety of insidious ways:

• Nicotine stimulates the release of epinephrine, which causes increased blood pressure and constricted blood vessels. If you've had a bypass graft and continue to smoke, the effect of nicotine in your bloodstream can close off the graft.
• Toxins in cigarettes injure the walls of the coronary arteries so that fat and cholesterol can be more easily deposited there. These poisons may increase your heart rate by as much as

twenty-five beats a minute and raise blood pressure by as much as twenty points.

• Cigarettes can cause blood clots, which can block already clogged arteries—this can trigger a heart attack.

• Cigarettes raise your LDL levels.

• Cigarettes can trigger coronary spasm, where the heart's blood vessels constrict and possibly damage the heart.

• Smoking may cause narrowing of blood vessels in the legs, kidney, and brain, a condition known as **peripheral vascular disease.** Symptoms of this condition include **claudication**— cramps in your calves when you walk even a short distance. It will be alleviated by rest but will start up again when you move.

In the Walnut Creek Study, smoking presented a threefold risk of heart disease in premenopausal women. How much you smoke makes a big difference in your risk, however. The risk of heart attack if you smoke fifteen to twenty-four cigarettes a day rises from 2.4 to 7 percent if you allow yourself over twenty-five cigarettes a day. The Nurses' Health Study, which tallied results from 119,000 women, showed similar dose-dependent findings for angina, heart attack, and deaths from coronary artery disease in women smokers.

SMOKING AND BIRTH CONTROL PILLS

If you smoke and also take oral contraceptives, you increase your risk drastically. The dosage of estrogen and progesterone in birth control pills tends to accentuate our body's tendency to form blood clots. This can lead to heart attack, stroke, or pulmonary embolism (a clot in the lungs). When you combine the risk of smoking (which also puts you in danger of forming blood clots) with oral contraceptives, you have a combined risk factor greater than either one taken individually. Comparing heavy smokers who didn't take birth control pills to heavy smokers who did, the risk rose from 4.8 to 23 percent!

Even if you don't smoke, you have an increased risk if you live with a smoker or spend time in a smoky environment. Inhaling passive smoke raises heart rate and blood pressure and increases your need for oxygen when you're exercising. The good news is that if you stop smoking, you can cut one risk factor in half after only one or two years. And after fifteen years of abstinence, there is no difference between an always nonsmoker and someone who has quit for good.

MULTIPLE PREGNANCIES

Women who have had five or more pregnancies—whether or not these result in live births—are at greater risk for heart disease. In a study done in England in 1989, women with five or more pregnancies had a .9 times greater risk of heart attack than women who had fewer pregnancies. Although women have higher levels of HDL during pregnancy (which is protective against heart disease), their HDL drops after delivery and remains lower than it was prior to conception. It's a good idea for women in this category to have their cholesterol levels checked frequently and, of course, to reduce other risk factors.

ALCOHOL

The medical world was rather surprised at the news from studies carried out in France that a couple of small glasses (four ounces each) of red wine each day would boost HDL levels and thus lower the risk of coronary heart disease. Does this mean that if you're a nondrinker you should begin to imbibe? Probably not.

It is true that a little alcohol may be beneficial, but the key word here is "little." One drink more a day begins to turn the picture drastically in the opposite direction—overconsumption of alcohol leads to liver damage, mental disorders, and increased risk of accident and injury. Women, also, can tolerate less alcohol than men not only because of their lower body weight but because they do not produce the same amount of stomach enzymes men do that process the alcohol and help to reduce its toxins.

If you do enjoy a glass of wine with your dinner, that's fine. But under no circumstances go overboard.

SOCIAL STATUS AND SOCIAL ISOLATION

We have many elements in our lives that seem out of our control. Where we sit in the social hierarchy—whether we are born in an urban ghetto or in a mansion—seems impossible to regulate. And our affinity for getting along with and spending time with others is also a rather indefinable category. Yet poverty and social isolation are two big risk factors for heart disease in women.

If you are poor, you tend to have less opportunity for higher education. Many high school dropouts who must go to work early to support a family simply never get back to school. Their lack of exposure to important information about preventive health care often stems from lack of funds to find and use health-care providers and lack of interest in or ability to read on their own. Since women are generally poorer than men in our society, a single woman without health insurance has a very hard time taking care of herself properly. She will undoubtedly be very sick before she is forced to seek medical care—and this may be through a visit to an emergency room after a heart attack.

As for social isolation, women here are also at a disadvantage. If you have no access to the support and warmth of a family, if many of your friends have died or moved away, if you aren't involved in community or neighborhood activities, you may be at higher risk for a variety of diseases. If you think back to Katharine's story, at the beginning of the chapter, you can understand better why feelings of loneliness and isolation might have contributed to her ambivalence about changing her lifestyle. It's hard to want to get better if no one is around to care whether you're well or sick.

What could Katharine, and others like her, do about these risk factors? If you are a poor woman but you are motivated to do something about your health, you certainly can. You can read on your own, attend adult education classes on preventive health care, and get yourself to a clinic for regular checkups.

If you are isolated and find it emotionally difficult to put yourself in social situations, you can relieve loneliness with a pet.

Documented studies show that touching and holding a dog or cat for a certain period of time each day relieves stress. The unconditional love you receive from an animal is rewarding to your sense of well-being. And if you have a pet dependent on you for food and daily walks, you have to stay well in order to take proper care of him. Walking the dog, as a matter of fact, is the one activity many couch potatoes favor—and the exercise is certainly beneficial!

How the Various Risks Affect Your Total Picture

As you can see, there are a lot of different factors here, but not all of them have equal weight. Looking at your situation as a whole, you will see that certain elements affect you much more than others. If you have a sick parent, an abusive husband, and have just lost your job, then stress is undoubtedly just as big a portion of your risk profile as your cholesterol count of 240 and the cigarettes you smoke each day.

It took you a while to accumulate your risks; it will take a while to reduce them. But whatever you do—just a little each day—will eventually have a huge impact on your heart health.

Risk Factor Quiz

Tally up the number of points and see where you stand. Although there are elements you cannot alter, you can subtract points for lifestyle changes you've consciously made. Remember that the *number* of risk factors is significant—independently, each risk is not as dangerous as a cluster of them added together.

If your score is 31–50, you are at high risk and should see a physician about making radical changes in your diet, exercise, and lifestyle.

If your score is 16–30, you are at medium risk, and could afford to make some small alterations in lifestyle.

If your score is under 15, you are in great shape! Keep up the good work!

1. How old are you?
   Ages 30–55   Add 1
   Ages 56–75   3
       75–100   4

2. Are you no longer menstruating? (either natural
   or surgical menopause)   Add 3

3. Did you have a close relative under the age of
   fifty-five with heart disease?   Add 4

4. Are you African-American?   Add 3

5. Are you diabetic?   Add 4

6. Do you sometimes neglect to take medications
   as prescribed?   Add 2

7. Do you smoke?   Add 4

8. Do you take birth control pills?   Add 4 if you
                                                       also answered
                                                       yes to number
                                                       7

9. Are you more than 20 percent over your
   recommended body weight?   Add 3

10. Do you never exercise?   Add 3

11. Does your diet consist of more than 30 percent
    of calories in fat?   Add 3

12. Is your blood pressure higher than 140/90 on a
    regular basis?   Add 2

13. Are your LDLs higher than 130?   Add 3

14. Are your HDLs lower than 45?   Add 3

15. Are your triglycerides higher than 200?   Add 3

16. Are you under a great deal of stress that you feel
    you can't handle?   Add 3

17. Do you feel lonely a lot of the time?   Add 2

18. Do you drink more than two glasses of alcohol
    (five ounces of wine or twelve ounces of beer)
    a day?   Add 2

19. Do you exercise daily?   Subtract 3

20. Do you eat mostly fruits, vegetables, and grains?   Subtract 3

21. Do you follow some specific program or pursue
    some personal activity that reduces your stress?   Subtract 3

22. Do you take replacement hormones?   Subtract 3

23. Do you drink one four-ounce glass of wine a day?   Subtract 1

24. Have you been a nonsmoker for at least five
    years?   Subtract 1

4

What to Eat for a Healthy Heart

∇

The expression "you are what you eat" isn't exactly on target. What is more accurate is "you *become* what you eat." After years of consuming certain foods and avoiding others, we do actually change the nature of our blood vessels, bones, brain, and internal organs. If we want to keep ourselves in wonderful physical condition, we have to *become* ever vigilant about what goes into our systems.

There is no pill or quick fix to wipe away suddenly the excesses of a lifetime. Food has a lot of emotional connotations for all of us—we nourish ourselves in adulthood with foods that make us feel comfortable, even if they're not particularly good for us. We can't change all our eating habits overnight, but we can make small changes over a long time.

In this chapter, we offer easy-to-follow graded steps to help you change the way you eat. By altering your diet, you can greatly lower the possibility of developing heart disease.

Medical science has not yet unraveled all the mysteries of the human heart—if we were all-knowing, we would be able to predict exactly which individuals would eventually get sick and designate those candidates for preventive care. We would earmark these people for special nutritional guidance, a personal trainer for the best cardiovascular workout imaginable, and a computer analysis of the various types of stress and the best methods to eliminate them.

But we don't know who is destined for heart disease. Any one of us, and certainly those of us with several of the risk factors discussed in Chapter 3, might develop angina tomorrow. And strange as it might seem, it's a good idea to consider ourselves candidates for heart disease because that concern will make us revamp many of the activities and choices we take for granted in our lives. We can actually *remove* some risk factors just by eating right and living a preventive lifestyle.

Nothing is impossible! Go slowly, at your own pace, and you will not only reduce your risks, but you'll enjoy life more.

Why Lifestyle Changes Are Beneficial to Your Heart

If you think about the progress of modern cardiac intervention, we have come very far indeed. Medical science has all kinds of amazing interventions and treatments—we can lower cholesterol and blood pressure with drugs; we can unclog arteries by expanding a tiny balloon against the cell walls; we can open the chest and actually repair the heart. However, these are strong medicine—sometimes so strong that they can do more damage than good, or even result in the death of the patient.

Women in particular are vulnerable when it comes to these interventions, which is why the preventive route becomes not just an option but an urgent answer. Yes, of course it is harder to change what you eat, how much you exercise, and how you live than it is to lie back and allow a doctor to "work" on you. But the results speak for themselves.

Not only can the proper lifestyle changes prevent you from having a heart attack or suffering from angina pain; they can actually reverse heart disease. Dr. Dean Ornish, a pioneer in cardiovascular care from the Preventive Medicine Research Institute in San Francisco, California, has shown that a plant-based, no-cholesterol diet combined with daily exercise and stress management can truly eradicate blockages in blood vessels and keep them clear. His patients are a testimony to the fact that human effort and simple, safe therapies that involve the most basic elements can save lives.

It didn't matter how old his patients were when they started—even arteries that had been blocked for years opened up on Dr. Ornish's program. Women as well as men saw excellent results. Understand, however, that Dr. Ornish's recommendations are stricter than the American Heart Association's—your diet must consist of only 10 percent fat, you must do some form of exercise each day, and you must also meditate, pray, or otherwise do some structured activity that will allow you to become calm and lower your blood pressure for at least half an hour a day.

If you are currently a healthy woman with a less than rigorous attitude toward nutrition, exercise, and stress, it is time to work on your preventive techniques. If you are already coping with heart disease, you have even more incentive to begin a careful program of lifestyle changes—with your doctor's supervision—that will enhance your medical treatment and keep you well.

Nutritional Strategies for Better Heart Health

"I never thought a minute about what I ate. I had one of those metabolisms that 'took a licking and kept on ticking,' " Adele, a sixty-one-year-old former schoolteacher, said. "My dad always grumbled about how I could eat an entire chocolate cake and *lose* weight, and it was true. The first-graders I taught used to joke about my mammoth lunches that spilled out of my lunch box.

"I never had any exercise program—nobody told me I was supposed to!—and I just loved fast food. For most of my life, my diet consisted of red meat, cheese, milk shakes, and candy bars.

"The year after I retired—I was 59—I was out mowing the lawn on a hot June afternoon when the pain hit. It felt like the lawnmower had jumped up on my chest. I guess that year I'd been much less active than I had when I was chasing my first-graders around, and the way I abused food finally got to my heart. The doctor said I had 85 percent blockages in two of my coronary arteries, and the third was 95 percent blocked. You can bet, after the bypasses, I was going to change what I put into my body. But you know, even now, even after two years of no meat or cheese, I can still taste that food in my head. That kind of food doesn't seem as appealing as it used to, even though I think about it sometimes. It's better to dream about it than let it kill you."

It's very clear—the more fat and cholesterol you eat, the more plaque on your arteries, the more danger to your heart. The *less* fat and cholesterol, the less plaque. (There are individuals who are predisposed to create an excess of cholesterol, no matter what they eat. However, most of us are able to adjust our LDLs and HDLs by modifying what we eat and how we move around.)

There is no reason why you can't learn to eat in a way that pleases you and also pleases your heart. But it must be learned and practiced—every day, at every meal. Most Americans consume a diet that gets about 40 percent to 50 percent of its calories from fat. Over years of eating this much fat, it would be unlikely *not* to develop blockages in our arteries. If you do not currently have heart disease, there is no reason why you can't manage your heart health on a diet that has 20 percent to 30 percent of its calories in fat. (In Chapter 11, we'll go over the more restrictive diet for those who have already had a heart attack or bypass surgery.)

The benefits you gain from healthy eating go way beyond protecting yourself from a heart attack. They will:

- Fill you with energy and well-being.
- Improve your body image as you see your shape changing to match your excellent eating habits.
- Motivate you to stick with an exercise program that will make you hungry for more good food.

The cycle of being healthy is self-perpetuating—one good habit feeds another. But you must cultivate the habits, first, before they can begin to alter your body and mind.

What to Eat

It is really rather simple if you use the U.S. Department of Agriculture food pyramid as a rough guide. But be aware! The recommendations of this pyramid are for a diet that takes 30 percent of its calories from fat, which is the absolute top amount you should be ingesting! If you have heart disease, you must stay at least 20 to 10 percent under its recommendations for fats and animal protein (which contain fats).

Food Guide Pyramid
A Guide to Daily Food Choices

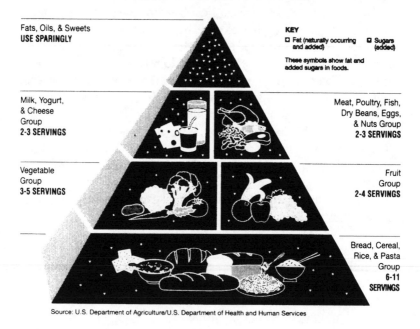

Fats, Oils, & Sweets
USE SPARINGLY

KEY
☐ Fat (naturally occurring and added)   ☑ Sugars (added)

These symbols show fat and added sugars in foods.

Milk, Yogurt, & Cheese Group
2-3 SERVINGS

Meat, Poultry, Fish, Dry Beans, Eggs, & Nuts Group
2-3 SERVINGS

Vegetable Group
3-5 SERVINGS

Fruit Group
2-4 SERVINGS

Bread, Cereal, Rice, & Pasta Group
6-11 SERVINGS

Source: U.S. Department of Agriculture/U.S. Department of Health and Human Services

You should be eating the proportion of your daily calories from the foods at the bottom where the pyramid is widest and increasingly less as you work your way to the pinnacle. For an *unrestricted low-fat diet,* you should be eating plenty of salad and cooked vegetables, fruits, legumes, fish and shellfish, poultry without skin, lean cuts of beef, lamb, pork, and veal; monounsaturated fats (canola and olive oils), some low-fat and fat-modified dairy products, and some fat-modified baked goods. You should consume:

- 50 to 60 percent of your daily calories in complex carbohydrates
- 20 to 30 percent of your daily calories in protein
- 20 to 30 percent of your daily calories in fats—lowering this percentage over time as you can.

For a good preventive care diet, you should be eating:

- *Bread, cereal, rice, and pasta:* six to eleven servings daily (Serving is one slice or half a cup.)
- *Vegetable group:* three to five servings of half a cup daily
- *Fruit group:* two to four servings of half a cup daily
- *Milk, yogurt, cheese group:* two to four servings, one cup each, low-fat varieties
- *Meat, poultry, fish, legumes, eggs and nuts group:* two to three servings. Meat, poultry, and fish serving is three to four ounces; legumes are half a cup; egg is one whole; nuts, approximately ten. *Eggs and red meat are more severely restricted on a preventive heart program* (see Eating, below).
- *Fats, oils, sweets group:* use sparingly. Best to restrict this group to a tablespoon of oil for cooking. See below for alternative suggestions to fats.

Shopping

This is the crux of the matter. If you buy the right ingredients, you can't eat the wrong meals. As long as your larder is stocked with the best of everything for your heart, you will be consuming the best. Unfortunately, the choices are not as easy as they used to be because supermarkets carry so many different products—a corn muffin can be higher in fat than a scoop of ice cream. So you have to know just what to choose as you go down the aisles.

How to Read a Label

Now that the FDA requires the food industry to come clean about their ingredients and food values, we have only ourselves to blame if we don't learn how to read the labels on every product. The new designations on all packaged goods *must* include vital information that will tell us all we need to know about what we're going to put in our mouths. Most prepared foods list their ingredients in descending order of the amount contained in the food. So if you pick up a package of store-baked muffins containing seven or more grams of fat per serving, and the first three ingredients are white flour, sugar, and eggs, don't take them home. You want to choose foods that are *low* in fat, sugar, and salt and high in fiber, complex carbohydrates, vitamins, and minerals.

Take a few minutes to familiarize yourself with the new food label on the facing page.

You must also look at the percentage of daily values to see how any food fits in your total consumption over a twenty-four-hour period. The commissioner of the FDA suggests that in order to eat healthfully, each item you consume should contain not more than 5 percent of your daily fat calories. Remember to select whole-grain, low-fat products, either homemade or store-bought.

The New Food Label at a Glance

The new food label will carry an up-to-date, easier-to-use nutrition information guide, to be required on almost all packaged foods (compared to about 60 percent of products up till now). The guide will serve as a key to help in planning a healthy diet.*

Serving sizes are now more consistent across product lines, are stated in both household and metric measures, and reflect the amounts people actually eat.

The **list of nutrients** covers those most important to the health of today's consumers, most of whom need to worry about getting too much of certain nutrients (fat, for example), rather than too few vitamins or minerals, as in the past.

The label of larger packages may now tell the number of calories per gram of fat, carbohydrate, and protein.

New title signals that the label contains the newly required information.

Calories from fat are now shown on the label to help consumers meet dietary guidelines that recommend people get no more than 30 percent of the calories in their overall diet from fat.

% Daily Value shows how a food fits into the overall daily diet.

Daily Values are also something new. Some are maximums, as with fat (65 grams or less); others are minimums, as with carbohydrate (300 grams or more). The daily values for a 2,000- and 2,500-calorie diet must be listed on the label of larger packages.

Nutrition Facts

Serving Size 1 cup (228g)
Servings Per Container 2

Amount Per Serving

Calories 260   Calories from Fat 120

	% Daily Value*
Total Fat 13g	**20%**
Saturated Fat 5g	**25%**
Cholesterol 30mg	**10%**
Sodium 660mg	**28%**
Total Carbohydrate 31g	**10%**
Dietary Fiber 0g	**0%**
Sugars 5g	
Protein 5g	

Vitamin A 4%	•	Vitamin C 2%
Calcium 15%	•	Iron 4%

* Percent Daily Values are based on a 2,000 calorie diet. Your daily values may be higher or lower depending on your calorie needs:

	Calories:	2,000	2,500
Total Fat	Less than	65g	80g
Sat Fat	Less than	20g	25g
Cholesterol	Less than	300mg	300mg
Sodium	Less than	2,400mg	2,400mg
Total Carbohydrate		300g	375g
Dietary Fiber		25g	30g

Calories per gram:
Fat 9 • Carbohydrate 4 • Protein 4

* This label is only a sample. Exact specifications are in the final rules.
Source: Food and Drug Administration, 1994

═══════════════════════════▽═══════════════════════════

The following health claims now have uniform meanings:

* The designation "low-caloric" means forty calories or fewer per serving.
* The designation "low-fat" means three grams or fewer per serving.
* "Fat-free" means fewer than 0.5 grams of fat per serving.
* "Low saturated fat" means one gram or less per serving.
* "Low-cholesterol" means twenty milligrams or fewer; and no more than two grams of saturated fat per serving.
* "Low-sodium" means no more than 140 milligrams per serving.
* "Sugar-free" means no more than 0.5 grams of sugar per serving.

═══

What Should Go into Your Shopping Basket?

BREAD, CEREAL, RICE, AND PASTA

* Buy whole-wheat products whenever you can because they're higher in fiber; stay away from white flour.
* If you're tired of bread, try bagels or flatbreads (packaged crackers, usually imported from Scandinavia). Stay away from buttery croissants, doughnuts, and pastries as well as store-made muffins, which are loaded with refined sugar, eggs, and white flour.
* Don't buy rice "mixes" with their own flavor packets. These are loaded with sodium. Instead, purchase plain brown rice in the bag.
* Experiment with different pastas—there are those made with spinach, beets, and carrots.
* Try the no-yolk noodles instead of regular egg noodles. The taste is practically identical.
* Be alert to all cereal labels: most prepared cereals are loaded with sugar and salt, and granolas (even low-fat varieties!) are high in fat. The best cereals are the plain bran varieties, which are high in fiber, low in sugar, salt, and fat.

VEGETABLE GROUP

You can eat as many of these as you like! Vegetables come in two varieties—starchy and nonstarchy. (Starchy includes potatoes, yams, squashes, and corn; nonstarchy includes everything else.)

• Fresh vegetables are always preferable. They can be steamed, baked, or eaten raw in salads.

• If you're buying canned vegetables, make sure they're the no-salt variety. Drain and rinse canned vegetables before cooking.

• If you're buying frozen vegetables, get the loose, dry-packed varieties. Don't buy the ones packed in sauces.

• If you love to garden, you can always make your own frozen vegetables by parboiling them after picking and putting them in the freezer. That way, you and your heart can enjoy summer bounty all year long.

FRUIT GROUP

Most fruits are wonderful for preventive heart health, and they're terrific when you're craving something to fill you up that has no fat or salt in it.

• Coconut is the only completely restricted fruit, because it's high in saturated fat (this goes for any product, sauce, or baked good made with coconuts or coconut oil).

• Avocados and olives are also high-fat. They're unsaturated, however, they are calorically dense, so keep your consumption to a minimum.

• Canned fruits are usually packed in sugary syrups and should be avoided; likewise commercially prepared applesauce.

• Frozen dry-packed fruits are fine for cooking and homemade milk shakes. Don't buy the ones packed in syrup.

MILK, YOGURT, CHEESE GROUP

This is one category on the pyramid that is the trickiest for those concerned about their heart's health. If you're modifying your diet, you will want to include fewer and fewer of these products in your meals over time.

• Stick with low-fat varieties at all times. Whole milk has 49 percent of its calories from fat; skim milk gets less than 1 percent from fat.

• Buy whipped low-fat cream cheese, which is airier and less dense than regular cheese.

• If you can't tolerate plain no-fat yogurt, you can add your own flavorings to it. A little honey and vanilla make a big difference. Be sure to buy yogurts with active cultures, which benefit your body by restoring friendly bacteria to your intestines.

MEAT, POULTRY

• Buy lean varieties of all meats and poultry.
• Take the skin off poultry; trim meat of all visible fat.
• Buy "select" instead of "prime" or "choice" cuts of beef—these tend to be lower in fat.
• Change the proportion of animal protein in your meals. Instead of thinking in eight-ounce portions, you will now think in three-ounce portions so that meat and poultry become side dishes instead of a main dish. You might try a Chinese stir-fry that's mostly vegetables and noodles with just a bit of meat thrown in for taste.
• Use ground turkey instead of meat in your meatloafs.
• Stay away from all processed meats at the deli counter—they contain about 70 percent of their calories in fat. This goes for chicken or turkey hot dogs as well.

FISH AND SHELLFISH

• Most fish and shellfish are good low-fat protein choices. Avoid very fatty fish, such as bluefish.
• Coho salmon, mackerel, albacore tuna, and rainbow trout are high in omega-3 fatty acids, which are helpful in reducing blood cholesterol.

• Don't buy frozen fish that's already breaded or covered with sauce.

• If you traditionally mix mayonnaise into your canned tuna fish, substitute low-fat mayo, or better yet, mix the tuna with a little vinegar or soy sauce.

LEGUMES

• Purchase loose-packed, dried beans. Chickpeas, black-eyed peas, lentils, as well as navy, black, mung, adzuki, garbanzo, kidney, and lima beans are excellent sources of protein.

• Beans and peas need to be soaked overnight or parboiled for a few hours before cooking in soups, stews, and main-dish casseroles.

• Beans do not necessarily cause gas. If you aren't used to having them in your diet, wean your way off animal protein and onto legumes slowly, starting off with smaller portions and working your way toward larger ones.

• Drain and rinse canned beans.

• Substitute tofu or tempeh for meat in your main dishes. These soy products that look like cakes of cheese and can be cooked in different ways seem to affect the heart positively for a number of reasons. They are relatively low in fat and also contain plant estrogens known as phytoestrogens. These may act like human estrogens in the body, binding to receptor sites in the cells to keep HDLs high and LDLs low.

EGGS

• One large egg yolk contains 275 milligrams of cholesterol, which is just about equal to the American Heart Association's daily allowance for cholesterol. This means that egg yolks are to be severely restricted, although the whites are pure protein and very good for you.

• Investigate egg substitutes, which you'll find in the freezer case of your supermarket. You must read the labels carefully, though, since those made with oil may equal a whole egg in fat calories.

* Make an omelet of egg whites and color it yellow with turmeric.
* Buy small or medium eggs and throw out one yolk for every two eggs.

FATS AND OILS
* Butter is very high in saturated fat and should be avoided completely for eating and baking.
* Margarines are not necessarily better for you because of their trans-fatty acids, but you can use them sparingly if you know what to buy. Margarine is made by treating oil so that it will "stand up" on a piece of bread. However, if it stands up too much, you're in trouble. The process known as "hydrogenation" takes liquid oil and turns it solid. How do you know what to buy? The first ingredient listed on the label is the major ingredient. So if you see "liquid vegetable oil" at the top of the list, you know you're buying a product low in saturated fat (high in polyunsaturates).
* Diet margarines are made with water and therefore a little goes a long way on a piece of bread. They are lower in fat than regular margarine but still generate trans-fatty acids, so they shouldn't be used liberally.
* Think about giving up butter and margarine for your bread completely and dipping lightly in olive oil, which is low in saturated fat.
* Avoid coconut and palm oils, which are high in saturated fats.
* Use polyunsaturated oils for cooking, especially corn oil. The best oils for lowering blood cholesterol cooking are monounsaturated—olive, canola, or corn oil.

SWEETS
* If you can do without, that's wonderful. Otherwise, use them sparingly and try to stay away from refined sugar.
* Eat sherbet or ices instead of ice cream.

• If you splurge on ice cream every so often, select the plain varieties rather than those loaded with chocolate chips, candy, or nuts.

SNACKS

Everyone gets the munchies. Make sure you have the following in the house:

• Air-popped popcorn.
• Raw vegetables (carrots, celery, peppers, mushrooms, zucchini, etc.) already cut and stored in glass jars in your refrigerator.
• Fresh fruit.
• Plain or low-fat yogurt.
• Fruit juice frozen into pops.

Cooking

Now that your refrigerator and cupboard is filled with good, nourishing foods, you have to know how to prepare them. You can enhance your excellent nutrition by using low-fat cooking methods. Here are some tips about all the different food groups:

BREAD, CEREAL, RICE, AND PASTA

• You can make your own breads by investing in a bread machine. This way, you get to use the best ingredients for your heart, and you also know exactly what's in every loaf.
• If you do your own baking, always substitute 2 percent milk for whole milk or cream.
• Make your own granolas with different grains and raisins.

VEGETABLE GROUP

• Vegetables can be baked, broiled, roasted, steamed, or poached. Don't boil them—water-soluble vitamins and minerals will vanish in the cooking water.
• You may also eat vegetables raw—this requires no additional fat and no nutrients will be lost in the cooking process. If you're sick of carrots, buy a juicer and make yourself carrot juice.

• If you feel vegetables are tasteless without a condiment, try lemon juice, soy sauce, chives, or salsa on top instead of butter or cheese.

FRUIT GROUP
• The best fruit is uncooked, but if you're cooking, don't use sugar. Toss with a fruit juice or a little honey.
• When you have a craving for pie, make your own with a wheat crust and fresh fruit with fruit juice instead of syrup to moisten it.

MILK, YOGURT, CHEESE GROUP
• In recipes that call for whole milk or cream, substitute skim milk thickened with cornstarch or evaporated skim milk.
• Substitute yogurt for sour cream.
• Substitute cottage cheese plus skim milk and a teaspoon of soft-tub ultra-low fat margarine for cream cheese.

MEAT, POULTRY, FISH, LEGUMES
• You can bake, broil, roast, steam, poach, or boil.
• Before you cook meat, trim off all visible fat and discard.
• Before you cook poultry, take off the skin and discard.
• When cooking legumes, add flavorings to your cooking water. You can use bay leaves, onion, garlic, and whatever herb will complement your recipe.

EGGS
• If a recipe calls for egg yolks or whole eggs, use one yolk and make all the rest egg whites. You can also use Egg Beaters or another egg substitute.

FATS AND OILS
• You should not fry, saute in fat, or dip foods in egg and batter before cooking them.
• You can occasionally use a small amount of monounsatu-

rated fats—olive or canola oil—in your pan to flavor your vegetables, legumes, or meats.

• Use a nonstick vegetable shortening spray (olive oil is best) to coat the pan.

• It is difficult to cook with the very low fat margarine products, mentioned above, because they also contain a great deal of water—use these (sparingly) for eating instead.

• You can "saute" vegetables and meats in a wok, using a small amount of broth, wine, or tomato sauce to moisten them.

• Don't buy commercial salad dressings. Make your own with olive oil and vinegar or lemon juice.

FLAVORING

• Cut down or cut out salt in your food preparation and at the table if you have high blood pressure.

• Experiment with herbs like dill, chives, parsley, taragon, curry, basil, and oregano in your cooking.

• There are also savory substitutes for salt (such as "Dash") that will add flavor to foods.

• You can use any of the following in preparation or at the table: lemon, mustard, ketchup, horseradish, salsa or taco sauce, vinegar, Worcestershire sauce.

EATING

This is the hardest part. You know what you've bought, you know how to cook it, but how do you make yourself consume only healthy foods all the time, every day, every meal, every snack?

WHAT DOES FOOD MEAN TO YOU?

Food is not like a vitamin pill or a special heart medication that you gulp down because it's good for you. Food implies nurturing and sharing with others. It can be a throwback to childhood, especially if you had the kind of mother who gave you a cookie if you felt sick, sad, or for no particular reason to express her love. Food is also a major component of socializing, mixing good conversation and laughter with enjoyable smells and tastes.

But you will have to change your attitude about food and love if you want to stay healthy. You will have to start convincing yourself that the cookie is a quick fix for your mouth; vegetables, fruits, and grains are the way you show your affection for yourself. And then you'll be able to rest easy about what effect the food you eat will have on your arteries.

THE MECHANICS OF EATING

Think of each meal as a holistic feast, a first supper rather than a last supper. In purchasing, preparing, and consuming foods that are good for you, you are indulging mind, body, and spirit. By taking in only those foods that will help your heart, you are doctoring yourself and truly taking charge of your body. Each morsel becomes a promise you make to yourself to stay well; each swallow another addition to the protective circle of health care you supply. This means, too, that you will no longer eat standing up or in front of the television. You will eat consciously, mindfully, thinking about what's going into you. Chewing each mouthful carefully will really allow you to taste food as you haven't in years; eating when you're hungry and putting down the fork when you're full will satisfy your brain and heart as well as your stomach.

GUIDELINES FOR GOOD EATING

Bread, Pasta, Cereal, and Rice Servings. One slice bread, ½ cup cereal, ⅓ cup cooked rice, or ½ cup pasta supplies 15 grams carbohydrate, 3 grams protein, a trace of fat, and 80 calories.

Vegetable Servings. ½ cup cooked or one cup raw supplies 5 grams carbohydrate, 2 grams protein, and 25 calories.

Fruit Servings. One whole fruit raw or ½ cup cooked supplies 15 grams carbohydrate, and 60 calories.

Meat and Legume and Cheese Servings. One ounce cooked meat/poultry/fish supplies 7 grams protein, about 5 grams fat, and about 75 calories. You may substitute one cup dried beans or peas or ½ cup tofu or one ounce low-fat cheese or one egg (limit two per week).

Milk Servings. One cup skim or 1 percent milk, or one cup plain low-fat yogurt supplies 12 grams carbohydrate and 8 grams protein.

Fat Servings. One teaspoon of polyunsaturated or mono-unsaturated oil, one tablespoon salad dressing or six dry-roasted almonds supplies 5 grams of fat and 45 calories.

KEEP AN EATING DIARY FOR A WEEK

Measuring food and counting calories can be boring and tedious. However, for the purposes of healing your heart, it is useful to see in black and white exactly what you eat each day.

The following meal plan, designed by dietitians at St. Francis Medical Center in Trenton, New Jersey, to help you in your eating choices, will make sense of the food pyramid. Since the biggest change you'll have to make in your diet is the amount of fat you consume, you will need a fat counter, which you can get at any bookstore and in many supermarkets and drugstores. Carry it with you, whether you're dining at home, in a restaurant, at a friend's house, or attending a wedding or special celebration.

Let's use an unrestricted diet of 2,000 calories a day as an example, since this is the amount gauged on commercial food labels. You know that no more than 30 percent of those calories (600) must come from fat. Since each gram of fat has 9 calories in it, you divide 600 by 9 to get your allowance of approximately 66 grams of fat per day. (Obviously, if you are trying to lose weight and are consuming fewer calories, you must do the arithmetic that pertains.)

Writing down everything you eat will make you conscious of the foods you put in your mouth. You can't cheat if you have to put pen to paper. If you do it for a week, you won't have to keep doing it if you're honest.

This diary should include everything you put into your mouth: the particular food, the amount, how it was prepared, and finally, the fat calories consumed. Compare at the end of the day with portions and types of food outlined on the food pyramid and see how you're doing. If your fat intake is too high for the first three days, resolve to do better for the rest of the week. The 30 percent allowance of fat calories is really pretty high for any woman concerned about her heart—although it's probably lower than what you're currently eating. Try to see if, at the end of the week, you can get those fat grams down to 60 or even 55 and to reduce the amount of red meat and junk food you are eating. The better you manage it, the more benefit to your heart.

What About Vitamin and Mineral Supplementation?

Controversies continue to rage over whether individuals who are eating a healthy diet need supplementary vitamins and minerals. In the case of heart disease, however, the prudent course is to supplement your good nutrition, particularly when it comes to antioxidants such as vitamins E and C, beta-carotene, and niacin (and other B vitamins), as well as calcium for strong bones.

Antioxidants roam through the body, scavenging for "free radicals," the wild chemical reactants that assist the destructive process of oxidation in a cell. Although our heart and bloodstream thrive on oxygen, it can be a destructive gas in the body when it gets out of control. The process of oxidation hardens the lens on the eye into a cataract, dries up the lubrication in our joints, and causes wrinkling of the skin. Because it helps to harden the arteries and make them less elastic, it is one of the chief culprits in heart disease.

If you supplement your diet with the right vitamins and minerals, however, you can thwart this process. Antioxidants deactivate free radicals and prevent them from forming branching chain reactions that can destroy the molecular structure of our cells. They can also help to strengthen cell walls so that free radicals can't invade.

Your Individual Meal Diary

BREAKFAST

Servings/Food Group	Type of Food	Portion Size	Preparation	Fat Content
__ Fruit				
__ Bread/cereal				
__ Milk				
__ Fat				
__ Other				

NOON

__ Bread/carbohydrate				
__ Vegetable				
__ Fruit				
__ Meat or legume				
__ Milk				
__ Fat				
__ Other				

EVENING

__ Bread/carbohydrate				
__ Vegetable				
__ Fruit				
__ Meat or legume				
__ Milk				
__ Fat				
__ Other				

SNACKS: (raw vegetables, salad greens, unsweetened dill pickles, air-popped popcorn, rice cakes, sugar-free gum, unsweetened cranberries or rhubarb.) _____

Daily Fat Grams _____

It is preferable to get our vitamins and minerals from the foods we eat, although in certain instances it is not possible to get *enough* of these elements from our diet. In those cases, we need supplementation. Note that the recommended daily allowances from the U.S. Department of Agriculture are much lower than the recommended amounts for antioxidant protection.

Vitamin C. (RDA 60 milligrams); recommended protective amount is 1,000 milligrams daily; food sources include broccoli, citrus fruits, tomatoes, and papaya. It is fairly easy to obtain all your vitamin C from food sources.

A report in the *American Journal of Clinical Nutrition* reported that the incidences of cardiovascular disease and cancer were lower in populations that consumed plenty of green leafy vegetables and fruit.

Vitamin E. (RDA 30 IU); recommended protective amount is 400 IU daily; food sources include olive oil, wheat germ, organ meats, and eggs. You will need supplementation, since it would be fairly difficult to get your daily amount from food sources without eating a great deal of fat.

Pigs on a diet high in vitamin E were found to have fewer myocardial infarctions. They were also able to recover from them more quickly than those that hadn't been given vitamins.

Beta-carotene. (no RDA); recommended protective amount is 6.6 milligrams daily or two carrots or one cantaloupe or two servings of squash. You can certainly get all the beta-carotene you need from food sources.

Though recent reports downgrade the effectiveness of beta-carotene in preventing lung cancer in chronic smokers, other studies underline its effectiveness. In a six-year study on 22,000 physicians, researched at Brigham and Women's Hospital in Boston, those who were given beta-carotene supplements as opposed to a placebo had fewer heart attacks, strokes, and other cardiac events. The Physicians' Health Study showed that eating foods that contain beta-carotene can reduce the risk of stroke, heart attack, and death from cardiovascular disease by one-half. This study showed that beta-carotene prevented the oxidation of cholesterol, which is not able to stick to artery walls when it is not oxidized.

Niacin (Vitamin B-3). (RDA 20 milligrams); recommended protective amount is 40 milligrams three times daily. Good food sources include meat, fish, poultry, milk products, peanuts, and brewer's yeast. You can probably get your daily required amount from food without supplementation.

This vitamin has been shown to have enormous success lowering LDLs and raising HDLs, particularly when administered in combination with a cholesterol-lowering drug such as Lovastatin. To avoid the typical "flush" that occurs when niacin is taken in large doses over a long period of time, an aspirin a day is also recommended.

Calcium. (RDA is 1,000 milligrams daily); recommended protective amount is 1,500 milligrams daily for women past menopause; 1,000 if they are taking replacement estrogen. Food sources are dairy products, green leafy vegetables, sea vegetables, and fish with bones. You may need supplementation unless you are willing to consume low-fat or nonfat dairy products or consume a great many sardines and green vegetables.

Calcium is indirectly helpful to the heart. It prevents bone loss and keeps bone density high, which means that a woman will be better able to keep up a cardiovascular exercise program because she won't be suffering from osteoporosis or untimely falls and fractures.

On top of the supplements recommended above, a good multivitamin once a day will round out your nutritional menu. A high quality supplement might include smaller amounts of the nutrients listed below. These are about two to three times higher than the U.S. RDAs:

Vitamin C—250 mg.
Vitamin E—150 IU
Vitamin A—7500 IU (one-half from beta-carotene)
Iodine—150 mcg.
Vitamin D—400 IU

Vitamins B-1, B-2, B-6, and Niacin—75 mg. each
Vitamin B-12—75 mcg.
Calcium—50 mg.
Potassium—10 mg.
Iron—10 mg.
Magnesium—7.2 mg.
Manganese—6.1 mg.
Zinc—15 mg.
Selenium—10 mcg.
Folic acid—400 mcg.
(Available as Formula VM-75 Tablets, Extra High Potency
Multivitamin from Solgar.)

Eating Out

Sandra, a fifty-five-year-old executive at a major corporation,
spent half her life eating prepackaged food on airplanes, and
then at business meetings, being plied with pastries at break time
and beef Wellington at lunch. Then she'd have a hotel meal
before retiring—usually something fast and easy like a cheese-
burger.

After her heart attack, she knew she couldn't continue this
way. "I sat down with my doctor and said, 'Look, I have to
travel, I have to eat, and I don't intend to carry a raw cabbage
and a bag of oat bran with me everywhere. So what do I do?'

"We took apart all the dangerous eating situations and figured
out options. For instance, the airlines will always give you a
vegetarian plate if you call in advance. And you can specify that
you want it steamed, not drowned in butter or smothered in
cheese sauce. The breakfasts were easy—eat the roll without the
butter and with a little jam occasionally. They generally also have
individual-size cold cereals, like raisin bran, that you can have
plain or with skim milk.

"The banquets were harder. I would always call in advance to
see if I could get a special plate; if I couldn't, I'd concentrate on
vegetables and rice or pasta on the plate and bypass the brisket

of beef or chicken Kiev. Since most of these functions take place in hotels, there's always a big fresh fruit basket around—sometimes if you're an honored guest they even put one in your room.

"If I was eating lunch with a client, again, we could sit around an office and order in from a deli, and I'd make sure to ask for an individual can of water-packed tuna or a big garden salad with dressing on the side. In restaurants, waiters are now used to taking very specific orders—no mayo, hold the sauce, broiled dry, etcetera."

As Sandra points out, the advantages of low-fat cooking and eating are not lost on the restaurant community. There are numerous eateries—from the most expensive elegant restaurants to comfortable family bistros—that serve "heart-healthy" meals. These are usually asterisked or marked by a heart in the menu.

If you don't happen to find yourself at one of these enlightened restaurants, you can select the most likely low-fat choice on the menu and then let the waiter (and the chef) know exactly how you'd like your food prepared:

- Baked, broiled, roasted, or steamed only.
- Salad dressing on the side.
- Vegetables cooked without butter.
- Pasta or rice with tomato-based, not cream-based sauces.
- Salsa instead of hollandaise, bearnaise, or any egg yolk–based sauce.
- An omelet made from egg whites.
- Fresh fruit cup only if the fruit is in its natural juices.

What's the Trick to Changing Your Way of Eating?

Think not of subtracting "bad foods" but rather adding "good foods." You should experiment with all sorts of fruits, vegetables, and grains you've never tried before. You should certainly eat more of foods that contain beneficial plant estrogens, such as tofu and tempeh and carotenoids such as carrots, apricots, mangos, papaya, squash, cantaloupe, pumpkin, and sweet potatoes.

Experiment with one new food or food preparation each week—even if you or your family members are picky eaters. If you keep adding new things and subtracting processed, high-fat, high-salt, high-sugar foods, you will all be on the right road to good nutrition.

Does low-fat shopping and eating mean that you can never again indulge in your favorite high-fat foods? That is a matter to discuss with your physician, and it completely depends on your psychological relationship to what you put in your mouth.

Some of us simply can't take deprivation—it causes so much stress to do without foods we love that our blood pressure rises and makes us sicker than we would have been if we'd eaten the ice cream or bacon. Every once in a while these individuals should eat what they desire.

If you truly love cashews, buy a jar and divide them into small packets of ten nuts apiece—or better yet, buy peanuts in the shells. Allow yourself a packet a week. Treat yourself to ice milk instead of ice cream once every two weeks.

If you feel you have no willpower at all and will not be able to live with forbidden foods in the house without consuming them all at one serving, don't buy them. If it is not in the house, you won't be able to eat it. Shop differently, and you will eat differently. If you are miserable with your daily diet choices as you begin to change your attitude toward food, you can always indulge your old cravings at a restaurant once a month or so, if your physician says it is all right. As long as you don't splurge on a regular basis, you'll be fine.

And if you modify the rest of your habits, you'll find heart-healthy eating to be much easier. The next chapter will open the door to other lifestyle changes—exercise, sleep, smoking cessation, and stress management—that will complement your new nutritional choices and help you to stick with them.

5

A Pound of Prevention:
Exercise, Smoking Cessation,
Stress Reduction, and a Good
Relationship with Your
Physician

▽

There are many roads to good health, and they all interconnect. If you're eating a good diet, but you don't get up and move around, you're defeating your own attempts at prevention. If you eat and exercise but leave your desk every break and lunch hour to puff on a cigarette, you are doing an incredible amount of damage to your heart. Exercise and smoking cessation can make an enormous difference in your heart-health profile when combined with an excellent program of nutrition. And when you add a dedicated stress-reduction program and a good relationship with a health-care provider who can see you through good times and bad, you have a prescription for a preventive-care program that can last you a lifetime.

So allow one good habit to spark another. Give yourself the benefit of total prevention, and you will be many steps ahead of the game when it comes to protecting your heart.

What Kind of Exercise—and How Much—Is Right for a Woman's Heart?

There is no question about whether exercise can reduce your risk of cardiovascular disease. Numerous studies have demonstrated clearly that an increase in physical activity is not only beneficial to your weight and lipid profiles, but it also reduces stress, thereby taking care of your heart simultaneously in many different ways.

In a study of five hundred women carried out over a three-year period around the time of their menopause—when their risk factors for heart disease were rising—it was found that the most active women had:

- lower weight
- lower systolic and diastolic blood pressures
- lower triglycerides
- lower LDLs and higher HDLs
- lower fasting and postprandial insulin levels.

Over a three-year span, the women who increased their exercise by only three hundred kilocalories per week (the equivalent of walking an extra three days a week for twenty-five minutes each time) did not see the same decline in physical or mental status as their more sedentary colleagues. It is expected that women passing through menopause will see a slight increase in weight and lowering of HDL cholesterol—but the exercisers didn't exhibit these problems. Exercise also helped to circumvent the depression that often strikes women at midlife—which may in turn cause them to abuse cigarettes or alcohol and thereby increase their cardiovascular risk.

A recent Johns Hopkins study examined arterial stiffness in men—and although the outcomes cannot immediately be extrapolated to pertain one for one to women, their dramatic results are significant. Male athletes (from fifty-four to seventy-five years old) who ran about thirty miles a week were compared to sedentary men and women and were found to have 30 percent less arterial stiffness, which is a primary cause of high blood pressure. What happens when we don't exercise is that the arterial walls thicken and the cells stop producing elastin, which keeps the walls flexible. When this happens, the arteries can't expand and contract with the blood flow that follows each heartbeat, and blood pressure rises.

But you don't have to be a marathoner to keep your arteries in shape. Another study divided subjects into five categories (from most fit to least fit) and found that the death rate was highest in the least fit but declined rapidly in the next category up. The second tier of female subjects who exercised only minimally had a death rate of 48 percent lower than those who did nothing at all. Just a brisk walk each day will make this huge difference.

Should you exercise more than you currently do? If you're not doing something physical every day, the answer is an emphatic yes. In addition to the positive changes to the body mentioned earlier, exercise promotes a better self-image and an elevated mood. These are qualities that serve us in good stead when we're thinking about taking the best care of our heart.

HOW DO I GET PHYSICALLY FIT?

Make yourself a schedule for progress and do a little more each week. It is essential to start slowly and work your way into activities that will stress your heart at an increasing rate. You are not aiming to knock yourself out or exercise so vigorously that you will injure yourself. It is much more important to do some moderate exercise every day than to overtrain several times a week. If you are a very healthy person when you start your exercise schedule, you will be attempting to raise your heart rate to a maximum rate calculated by this formula:

$$220 - \text{your age} \times 70 \text{ percent.}$$

For example, if you are 50 years old, it would be $220 - 50 = 170 \times 70$ percent $= 119$.

If you are recuperating from a heart attack or have already been diagnosed with heart disease, 70 percent may be too high. Your physician must prescribe the correct percentage for your ability.

It's very simple to learn how to take your own pulse. Just count the number of heartbeats by feeling the pulse in your neck or wrist for fifteen seconds, then multiplying by four. Do this first at rest, then after you've been exercising for about twenty minutes, then as you recover. As you get into better shape, you'll find that your heart rate gets back to its normal resting rhythm more quickly.

You are aiming for an aerobic fitness level that will improve the pumping action of the heart muscle. When you exercise, your muscles demand more oxygen. Naturally, they get this oxygen as it is carried in the blood. As you inhale deeply during strenuous exercise, your heart beats faster and contracts more powerfully. Over time, your heart accommodates to the new demands put on it and is able to recover more quickly when you relax after exercising. This means that the heart—and the arteries and veins that supply it with blood—becomes more efficient as you work out more.

Aerobic fitness, however, doesn't equal total fitness. In order to have overall "competence" as an exerciser, and to do your heart the most good, you have to work on flexibility, endurance, and muscle strength as well. This means that it is a good idea to mix and match your exercise regimens—and if you don't do the same thing day after day, you can't get bored.

A nice mix would be:

- walking with hand weights for aerobic fitness plus
  tennis or racquetball for strength plus
  taijiquan (tai chi chuan) for flexibility and endurance, or
- walking for fitness plus
  biking for endurance plus
  yoga for flexibility, or

* stretching for flexibility,
  swimming for endurance plus
  monitored weight training for strength plus
  low-impact aerobic, or folk, or square dancing for aerobic
  fitness

One way to become physically fit is to change your mind about having to become a "jock." Many women are scornful of getting hot and sweaty because they were brought up to be good, clean little girls. But it takes sweat to work the heart, and every woman—regardless of her age, health status, or family history—has to work that muscle along with all the other muscles. If you don't use it, you lose it.

When you start thinking of exercise as a positive cardiovascular benefit, you can see that you don't have to knock yourself out—you don't have to become a marathoner or power lifter. It takes a long time to build up stamina and expertise in whatever exercise mode you choose—but by doing so, you build in more healthy years on your life span.

So take your time. Consult your doctor about what and how much you can do. Get yourself a good pair of walking or cross-training shoes. Progress a little every week, every month, every year. Never stop—because that's the way to keep your heart in shape.

HOW DO I AVOID EXERCISE BURNOUT?

It is very difficult to keep to an exercise program, particularly if you've never done it before. The general pattern is to start out enthusiastic—sometimes so much so that you throw yourself into the fray and sustain an injury. Then as you recuperate and can't perform the same activities, you lose your spur to exercise daily. It is just too much trouble to get up earlier or stay out later; it is too hard and only feels good when you stop. And then the regimen comes to a grinding halt.

In order to prevent this, you *must* make a written commitment to yourself.

The Unbreakable Exercise Promise

For the health of my heart, and the well-being of my mind and body, I agree to (1) get up half an hour earlier or (2) take half an hour before lunch or dinner, or (3) take half an hour before bed and do some form of physical exercise. This activity may be a daily walk, a period of stretching, an organized sports activity performed alone or with a friend, or a visit to a gym or health club to exercise, swim, or take a class.

I promise myself that I will perform some physical activity every day unless I am sick or injured, in which case I will return slowly to my exercise regimen after my recuperation.

I promise that I will look at this commitment as a gift to myself, a way of healing both my heart and my mind.

Signed, _____

(fill in your name)

Aside from your organized exercise schedule, there are many things you can do to increase your activity level without taking any extra time from your day.

- Walk or bike to your destination instead of driving.
- Park several blocks away from your destination and walk the rest of the way.
- When you take your children or grandchildren to the park, play with them instead of sitting on a bench and watching.
- Take the stairs instead of the elevator or escalator.
- Throw away your remote control—get up to change television channels.
- Put a piece of exercise equipment—a treadmill, rowing machine, StairMaster, or exercise bike—in front of your television and always use it when you watch a program.

Stress and Women: If You Can't Cut Out, Cut Down

Why are we so stressed out? Why are women in particular unable to calm their minds and relieve the pressure of daily concerns? There are, of course, type A women who are quick to anger, aggressive in the pursuit of their goals, and impossible to please.

But these women, like the type A men who were initially studied as being at high risk for heart disease, may in fact handle their stress *better* than most of us. They thrive on the challenge and excitement of looking at a bad situation, wrestling with it, and quelling it. Because type A's tend to see stress as an immediate issue that can be dealt with, they are not in terrible jeopardy of doing damage to their heart.

Those who can't see an end to the stress, however, are those in most peril. Prolonged, protracted, unalleviated stress is the kind that raises LDL cholesterol as it pumps in the stress hormones that may cause negative changes in the blood vessels. Those who take on the burdens of job, home, and everything in between have been designated as "type E" women by psychologist Harriet Braiker in her book, *The Type E Woman*.

Type E women often feel responsible for everyone else's problems—their partner's, their children's, their elderly parents', their boss's, their friends'. The incredible burden that a woman can shoulder is never acknowledged, and rarely do we get any thanks for fitting all this incredible emotional *sturm und drang* in our lives. Yet the constant pressure, the necessity to perform well, the craving to be perfect, have sent many a woman to the emergency room. What happens is that the "fight or flight" response never gets closure—the tightened muscles, the knot in the stomach, the arteries that constrict, in effect, to "hold on to" the blood should danger arise, just don't go away. And when arteries narrow, blood clots can form, spasms can occur, and heart attacks can happen.

If you are never satisfied with what you do or with what anyone else does—on the job or at home—you will never have the luxury of lowering your stress hormones. In tests done on men and women in the workplace, it was found that men's stress hormone level plummeted as soon as they left the office and were headed back to their families. Women's stress hormone levels, however, remained high when they arrived home—because home for most women is a second job.

Even in situations where the men were active participants in the management of the household, the woman was still overseeing most of the homework. Men's home tasks, from child care to lawn mowing to doing the checkbook, had no time constraint. However, women's tasks, from shopping to cooking to chauffeuring kids to classes to child-care emergencies, all had to be performed by a certain time. The pressure was on, day and night.

HOW TO LOOK AT STRESS WITH A NEW EYE

You have to admit that you've got a problem before you can begin to solve it. Here are some tips for analyzing your own stress situation:

• Each time you feel overwhelmed, stop and figure out exactly what it is that's causing your stress. When you are aware of what pushes your buttons, you can either try to avoid it or deal with it differently.

• Prioritize your stresses. Even if you feel they're all equally burdensome, you can only deal with one at a time. Pick the most mammoth, and let the others go while you handle it. Then move on to the next and so forth.

• Abandon your concerns about things that are completely out of your control. Let someone else take care of them.

• Delegate responsibility, both at work and at home. No, the jobs will not be done exactly as you would do them. But you will learn to appreciate others' competence as you learn to lower your impossible standards for perfection.

• Rally support for what you do and who you are. This can be an informal group of friends you call when you feel overwhelmed, or a formal group that meets every few weeks or so.

PROVEN METHODS OF RELIEVING STRESS

When we don't cope effectively with all the many things that bother us, our constantly elevated stress hormones and blood pressure put a considerable burden on our hearts (see Chapter 3). Exercise itself is stress reduction for many, and it works in a wonderfully efficient way to lower stress hormones and produce a natural high—a physiological phenomenon that occurs when the brain manufactures substances known as beta-endorphins, which act as natural opiates to relieve pain and anxiety.

Many women interviewed for this book said that they were able to calm their mind as they ran by the river with their dog, took an invigorating bike ride in the country, or concentrated on a good game of tennis with a friend. The experience of letting the mind float free without any particular focus is a typical one for many swimmers and runners.

But not everyone is able to forget the frustrations and anxieties of the day as they exercise. For many, an organized program of stress reduction is necessary.

There are several excellent methods of relieving stress.

Prayer. Those who have a strong belief in a power greater than themselves say that there is nothing like prayer to settle the spirit. Particularly for women who come from a religiously observant family, this modality of attentive awareness is extremely useful. While saying a rosary, reciting a psalm, or silently offering up positive thoughts, you are able to clear your mind of unpleasant worries and difficulties.

Meditation. Similar to prayer, the various types of meditation are comforting methods of quieting the mind. The idea is not to remove all stimulation but rather to concentrate on one sound, one word, one image, or one's breath for a protracted time. Herbert Benson, M.D., a professor at Harvard Medical School, who coined the phrase "the relaxation response," found that blood pressure was lowered, heart rate slowed, and muscle tension decreased during meditation. He also documented the fact that oxygen needs of the body are lessened during meditation and that arrhythmias are not as frequent. "Mindfulness meditation," where you focus your attention on one thing you are currently doing, is an easier practice for many novice meditators.

Jon Kabat-Zinn's excellent book on the subject, *Full Catastrophe Living*, outlines this technique.

Visualization or Guided Imagery. This specific healing technique asks the practitioner to imagine her illness in terms of a concrete object and change it in her mind. If you have a valve malfunction, for example, you might think of the leaflets of that valve as swinging doors, opening and shutting in a regular rhythm. If you have coronary blockages, you might imagine a tiny drill, working its way through the fatty deposits in your arteries, gently clearing the path. With this technique, you empower yourself to relieve the source of illness mentally. Studies have shown that cancer patients who used guided imagery in addition to their chemotherapy were able to reduce the size of their tumors over a six-month period faster than those who used no imagery and only chemotherapy.

Biofeedback. This technique teaches you to alter involuntary bodily processes with the aid of a monitoring machine. By manipulating signals you get from the machine, you can learn to release muscle tension, lower blood pressure and heart rate, or change your body temperature.

Sensors running from the machine are attached to your skin and give readings of your vital signs. By focusing mentally and physically, with the help of a trainer, you can alter the readings. By thinking angry thoughts, you can raise blood pressure; by thinking calming thoughts, you can lower it. One of the best uses of biofeedback is to manage stress by gaining control over physical elements that have exacerbated your tension. Your doctor may be able to recommend a qualified trainer, or you can get a referral from the American Association of Biofeedback Clinicians, located in Des Plaines, Illinois.

Self-hypnosis. This form of meditation allows you to sink deeper into your consciousness and alter your physical and emotional receptivity. With practice, you can put yourself into a state of calm and equanimity and give yourself suggestions that will change your physical state. You may wish to tell your heart that it is a lyrical singer, keeping perfect time with the orchestra.

You may want to suggest to a narrowed artery that it is opening and expanding like a garden hose with water coursing through it. Some psychiatrists and psychologists are trained in hypnotherapy. Ask your doctor or check with a local university hospital for a referral.

Yoga. Yoga is a series of postures, or asanas, that are held for different periods of time as you breathe into all parts of your body. This ancient Indian practice has been used successfully in many cardiac rehabilitation programs. Dr. Dean Ornish of the Preventive Medicine Research Institute in San Francisco, feels that yoga has been one of the linchpins of his successful stress-management program. The practice of yoga keeps the *prana,* or body's energy, in balance, which in turn keeps the entire cycle of mind and body in balance.

Tai Chi. This Chinese form of moving meditation offers not only a calm awareness of the spirit but the additional benefit of a flexible, strong body. The word *chi* means the same as *prana.* The purpose of learning the graceful tai chi exercises or forms is to move the energy stored in the body to promote health and longevity. The Taoist philosophy behind these movements stresses the need for balance of yin and yang, which comprise all the yielding and the forceful elements in life. Both yoga and tai chi are often taught at Y's and health clubs, and there are many corporations that now offer classes in these as lunchtime options for stress management.

Support Groups. There are support groups for nearly any problem you have to deal with—you can usually find them in the yellow pages of your local phone book under "Social Service Groups," "Women," and "Health." Your local hospital may also run a Heart Healthy program—ask your doctor or call the hospital social worker. If you can't find a group, start one yourself. The importance of having others around you who share your concerns cannot be overestimated. Women in isolation, keeping their problems to themselves, are at high risk for cardiac events, which is why meeting with a sustained group of those who care is so important.

STRESS QUIZ

How do you know if you're stressed? Take the following quiz and answer all questions honestly.

1. Are you a "take-charge" person?
2. Do you feel that you always have to be in control of a given situation?
3. Do you find it difficult to take criticism or follow directions?
4. Do you feel that your work is never done?
5. Are you a worrier? Does every little thing bother you?
6. Do you make everyone else's problems your own?
7. Do you ever take time for yourself?
8. Do you take on more tasks than you can possibly accomplish?
9. Do you rush from one activity to the next without allowing time in between to let things filter down?
10. Do you eat quickly?
11. Do you finish other people's sentences for them?
12. Do you find it difficult to keep quiet and listen to others?
13. Does it take you a long time to fall asleep at night?
14. Do you get unreasonably angry at other drivers on the road?
15. Do you find it unbearable to wait on line?
16. Do you put off responsibilities until the last minute, then race to meet a deadline?
17. Are you impatient with other people's slowness or deliberateness?
18. Do other people often disappoint you?
19. Do you try to plan most of your children's activities rather than allow them to decide what they want to do?
20. Do you feel it necessary to "fix" things immediately in your marriage or work situation instead of letting them come to their natural conclusion over time?

If you answered yes to fifteen or more questions, you are under a great deal of stress and should begin some stress-reduction program or technique. If your score is ten or less, you should make a concerted effort to structure some quiet time—prayer, meditation, yoga, or tai chi class—into your week.

LIFESTYLE CHANGES

We do terrible things to ourselves in the name of expediency, or for a certain type of pleasure, or because others do it and we want to be like them and liked by them, or because we need some outlet for our stress and no one has shown us a better way to relieve tension. The habits we create over a lifetime may be destructive, but they serve a purpose—they give us moments of respite from parts of our life too intolerable to confront.

So we smoke cigarettes, drink alcohol, indulge in recreational drugs, live in polluted, crowded cities, and deprive ourselves of healthful sleep each night. All of these lifestyle choices are exceptionally harmful to the heart.

In Chapter 3 we discussed risk factors that increase the likelihood of developing coronary artery disease—it is very clear that cigarettes and drugs (of which alcohol is one when overused) can bring on a variety of physical symptoms. But what is more dangerous even than the effects of nicotine, tars, and ethanol on the heart is the emotional dependency on these substances that keeps the habits alive.

Women are conditioned to cover their anger and tension—to explode or confront an attacker is considered "unladylike." And this is the reason that more women are closet drinkers as well as overeaters. Smoking, although it has decreased in the male population, is epidemic among young women these days.

Women would rather avoid stress than deal with it—lighting a cigarette, popping open a beer, or puffing on a joint can dull the pain or frustration for a while. But these palliatives offer no solutions to any problems. Instead, they damage the body as they dull the spirit.

Lack of sleep or living in a polluted, crowded area aren't exactly parallel to the other habits we've mentioned, but they, too, wreak havoc on a woman's heart. It was found that rats that were crammed into cages with no privacy and no "turf" of their own, in an environment where they had to fight for every morsel of food and even space to lie down, were more prone to develop mental and physical illnesses and to die at younger ages. Deprived of rest, they couldn't ever really relax, and they never reaped the benefit of the deeper levels of healthful, restorative sleep—the time when the body's hormonal activity can work overtime for healing and regrowth.

Not all of us can afford a country house or even a summer at the shore. And naturally, there are times when we have so much to do that we don't get enough sleep. But we owe it to ourselves to make some simple lifestyle changes that will make a difference in our heart health.

PROGRAM FOR LIFESTYLE CHANGES

1. Smoking. If you are a smoker, get into a program and stick with it. Offer yourself rewards at various stages to keep yourself on track. Smoking is one of the more insidious addictions, as we have learned from the recent media exposure about tobacco manufacturers. This means that to kick the habit, you must work at it during every waking moment and make sure you have plenty of support.

Here are some more tips to help you quit:

• When you feel like a cigarette, chew sugarless gum, have a glass of water, or eat a carrot stick.

• Keep away from situations where you tend to light up—if having a cup of coffee is your trigger, switch to tea, and eventually to herbal tea or a roasted grain beverage that tastes like coffee. If you always smoke when you're on the telephone, make sure you have a pencil and pad to play with as you talk.

• Don't hang out with friends who are smokers—or ask them not to smoke when you're around.

• Your doctor may be able to prescribe a nicotine patch or Nicorette gum for you, but these aids will only work when used in combination with a smoking-cessation program. The mechanical tools for quitting are just that—you will have to change your mind before you can change your habits. Most smokers know that smoking is bad for them but feel they haven't got the willpower to do anything to help themselves. A good program will keep you honest and motivated to stop, and the counselor and others in the program with you will help to keep you on track with your good intentions.

• Join a support group. This can be one of the most useful tools for maintaining a new and difficult pattern of self-care.

2. Alcohol. If you overuse alcohol or abuse recreational drugs, don't buy the products anymore. If it is not in the house, you won't be able to use it. Don't spend time with friends who drink or use drugs. Try switching to nonalcoholic beer (it contains .5 percent alcohol, but a couple of these a day will not have any impact on your heart). It is more common for women to drink alone, at home, but if you have always enjoyed the company of others when you drink, stay away from bars. It may be difficult for you to order a soft drink or a seltzer if you're with other people who are drinking alcohol.

3. Sleep. Change your sleep habits gradually. Make sure you are tired at night (moderate daily exercise will ensure that you get a good night's rest), and don't nap during the day—a common problem of older people who may not have to follow a schedule or go to an office. A cup of warm milk whirred up in a blender with a banana (both contain tryptophan, an amino acid that promotes sleep) really does do the trick at night—forget the sleeping pills, on which you can become too reliant. If you typically go to bed late, try retiring fifteen minutes earlier each night, and set the alarm clock for a specific time in the morning. If you go to bed at a reasonable hour but can't fall asleep, try some quiet breathing, which will allow you to relax. Even if you don't get down to the deeper layers of sleep, breathing will induce a meditative state that settles the mind and refreshes the body.

4. Environment. If you live in a crowded, busy city, make your own respite. It may be a weekend trip to a certain park where you can sit quietly and contemplate a tree or some flowers. It may be a subway ride to a beach where you can sift through the sand and walk in the waves. You can also create a "quiet room" for yourself at home—a place without distractions, telephones, or obligations—where you can sit for half an hour a day and think, pray, listen to soft music, or stroke your cat. One great tool for management of environmental stress is a long, hot bath.

These changes will not be easy, nor will you feel their benefit immediately. But they are essential if you are to stay healthy and even more vital if you are recuperating from a cardiac event.

Your Relationship with Your Health-Care Provider

It is very difficult to find a physician who is competent in the *human* realm as well as the medical, one who can guide the course of a discussion about big issues like lifestyle modification, health behaviors, anxiety, illness—even life and death. What you want from your doctor is an informed opinion and a sensitive ear. At the end of your appointment, both doctor and patient should feel they have gotten their points across. By talking and listening appropriately, coming together from a position of mutual respect, doctor and patient can work together for a good outcome.

Ask and you shall be given better health care. *Ask and keep asking.* Learn the right questions to ask and how to frame them so that they're direct but tactful. If you're not confrontational or docilely accepting, you can get what you need from your physician. If you're uncertain about what to ask, do some research on your own about your heart. Read books like this one and look for articles by competent journalists on your particular condition.

It is sometimes hard to ask your doctor just what you want to know. You may feel rushed or confused, or physically unwell and not really motivated to do any work yourself at the interview. You just want to be examined and taken care of. But you can't be a passive patient—not if your goal is the best heart health available.

It is your responsibility to help your physician learn everything she can about your condition. "Just what the doctor ordered" doesn't work anymore as a treatment option. If you are going to take control of your health care, you aren't going to accept "orders" from anyone. Instead, you're going to foster a give-and-take relationship with the physician or other health-care provider you see. If you don't think of your doctor as the ultimate authority but rather as a guide to better health care, your chances for a good outcome will improve immediately.

HOW TO TALK TO YOUR DOCTOR SO SHE WILL LISTEN
1. Give as much information *before* you see your doctor as you can. Fill out the office questionnaire honestly and completely and talk to the nurse or aide who interviews you in the waiting room.
2. Describe your symptoms clearly and directly, without apologies. Be as specific as you can about the activities that bring on pain or discomfort.
DON'T SAY: "You'll probably think I'm neurotic, but whenever I get nervous, I get this pain in my chest. It's probably nothing."
DO SAY: "I've been having this disturbing pain in my chest for the last three weeks. I'd like to find out if it's angina, and if so, what's causing it."
DON'T SAY: "My energy is completely gone. I feel so blue and depressed I can't make my regular tennis date."
DO SAY: "I have a weekly tennis date and I've never missed one in the past two years. But these days I get so short of breath when I return the ball, I've almost decided to quit playing, and just the thought of that depresses me."
3. Make some notes about what you want to say to the doctor before you go to your appointment and take them with you.
4. Consider taking a spouse, friend, or relative with you to the examination. If you are anxious about your condition, you may not hear exactly what the doctor is saying, and this may make you unable to respond. A companion in the examining and

consultation rooms can make a big difference in the kind of respect and attention you receive.

5. If this is your first appointment, pay attention to the way the physician responds to you. Remember, you are a paying customer, and you deserve good service. Does the doctor listen when you speak or does she interrupt? Does she answer the questions you've asked or admit she doesn't know but she'll try to find an answer? When she examines you physically, how comfortable do you feel? Think about the ways in which she asks you to do certain things—to move, to cough, to open your gown for further examination. She should still be attentive to your needs even while she assesses your condition.

6. Answer honestly when the doctor asks you questions. Tell her what your diet and exercise schedule are like and whether you smoke or drink. List all your various medications—both prescribed and over-the-counter—and explain why and when you take these drugs.

7. Be as specific as you can when talking about your pain (where it is, how often you experience it, what kind of pain you feel), shortness of breath, nausea, palpitations, or any other symptoms you've noticed.

8. Don't accept "you're just depressed and overtired" as a diagnosis. Don't accept a prescription for antianxiety medication as a substitute for a thorough cardiac workup. If your physician refuses to take your symptoms seriously, consult another doctor.

9. Listen to the doctor's responses and to her assessment of your health status without being defensive or guilty. Remember that you are partners in the process of getting you well, so be open to any changes she may suggest in lifestyle or health behaviors. Pay close attention to her advice about future testing or a change in medication. It's a good idea to take notes so that you can review what was said between you later.

10. Be sure that you understand the diagnosis and recommendations for treatment. If you don't know why you should be having a certain test or taking a certain medication, ask. You

might want to know if there is an alternative to an invasive procedure, or whether the amount of stress you're having influences the way your body behaves. If you need more information, request an article or a book to read on the subject.

11. Never spring another ailment or set of symptoms on your physician at the end of the examination. It may be tough to talk about what's really bothering you, but you will get much better care and more respect from your doctor if you list all your concerns at the start of the appointment, in descending order of importance to you.

12. Find out how the doctor will communicate with you in the future (for test results) and how and when you can best get hold of her. Be sure you know how you can reach your doctor in an emergency, especially on weekends and after hours.

13. If you have a condition that necessitates care by more than one doctor, find out how your primary care physician will coordinate your care by various specialists.

14. If you are being treated for heart disease, be prepared. Though you may never suffer a heart attack, it is best to establish a plan of operation with your doctor that can go into effect if you are incapacitated. When you have your wishes about treatment in writing, you can get prompt and appropriate attention from ambulance personnel as well as in the emergency room. (See Chapter 10 for a detailed description of this plan.)

15. Find out who covers for your doctor on vacation and ask any relevant questions about the other physician's credentials and experience.

16. Be sure you understand the way your physician handles payment. Her nurse or office administrator will be an invaluable aid in this area.

Being up-front with your physician is essential to feeling better sooner, because by dealing openly with her, you will be giving your health-care practitioner the tools she needs to provide you with better service.

Prevention Is Worth It

You may not feel that the suggestions for diet, exercise, stress management, and lifestyle changes are appropriate right now. You feel just fine, your last checkup was perfect, and you don't see any reason to alter the comforting rituals of your life.

But the point to make about prevention is that it doesn't show. You can't see the benefits right away—although if you stick with the program, you will feel and look 100 percent better than you ever have. If you want to keep your heart in excellent shape in the years to come, you have to start now.

6

Hormone Replacement Therapy: Is It Right for You and Your Heart?

∇

If you're postmenopausal and no longer have the protection afforded to your heart by the estrogen your body used to produce during your menstrual cycle, should you take replacement hormones to lower your risk of heart disease?

If there was a simple answer to this question, women past menopause would rejoice. But unfortunately there are no definitive answers. Hormone replacement therapy (HRT) is a boon to some women; not to others. Only you and your physician together will be able to decide what's right for you—and then you'll both have to leave the door open in case it is advisable for you to change your minds several years down the road.

Charlotte, at fifty-one, is a trim, active woman who runs her own business. She's a former smoker who now scrupulously avoids getting in the way of anyone else's smoke. She walks regularly, but her work schedule is so unpredictable, she ends up skipping meals and then bolting down food when she can. "I assumed I had indigestion when one day, after gulping a sandwich, I had terrible chest pains and tingling down my left arm. But when the pain kept coming back, I finally made an appointment to see a cardiologist.

"According to my ECG, that was no stomachache—that was a heart attack! Why did I suddenly get sick? Well, I was under incredible stress—my husband's business was in trouble at just about the time I started my own company. And there's a family history too—my mother had heart and lung disease (both heart failure and emphysema).

"Anyhow, I came out of it okay, and my doctor put me on medication. But our biggest discussion was all about hormones. I was exactly the right age to take them, and I'd been having hot flashes like crazy. The doctor said I was a particularly good candidate for replacement hormones because, first, the best statistics on reducing risk with hormones are for women who've already had a heart attack. I'd also had a hysterectomy a few years earlier. That meant I could just take estrogen [ERT as opposed to HRT] and get all the benefits for my heart without the drawbacks of the progestin. I've learned that in addition to taking care of my cholesterol, the estrogen is improving my endothelial tone—that means the insides of my blood vessel walls are more elastic and in better shape than they were.

"I'm still not sure I want to stay on the therapy forever. The idea of taking this for the rest of my life worries me because of the possible risk of breast cancer for long-term users. But my doctor said nothing's carved in stone—I can always change my mind."

Why Are Replacement Hormones Recommended to Postmenopausal Women?

During our reproductive years, our rhythmic menstrual cycle is testimony to our good hormonal health. Our brain sends out chemical messages to our ovaries, which in turn produce estrogen and progesterone on a fluctuating basis—estrogen governs the first half of the cycle, and then, after an egg has ripened and pushed its way out of the ovary in the process known as ovulation, progesterone governs the second half.

Estrogen is an enormously important hormone to the female

heart—and to the body in general. Since estrogen raises the HDL levels of our cholesterol and keeps the LDL levels low, we know that our hearts will be protected from plaque deposition during our reproductive years. Estrogen receptors help to keep blood vessel walls elastic and flexible, thus ensuring that blood pumped from the heart will flow smoothly through arteries and veins. Estrogen is also responsible for the health of over three hundred of our body's tissues. Its presence ensures that the genitalia will remain elastic and lubricated, that the skin will keep its youthful unlined glow, that our bones will retain their mineral content and keep substantial mass and density. Because estrogen interacts with the beta-endorphins in our brain—those neuropeptides that give us a sense of well-being—we are blessed with a generally positive outlook on life.

After menopause, however, when our menstrual cycles cease, the production of estrogen drops to within 20 percent of its former high. Although our fat cells are able to help out and produce a weakened form of estrogen called estrone, we are no longer in the safe haven of hormonal protection and are at the mercy of a variety of body processes. We may experience hot flashes as our brain hormones struggle to get our temperature in balance, we may have vaginal dryness that makes intercourse difficult or painful, and we may find that our cholesterol level begins to rise as the ratio of HDLs to LDLs begins to drop.

This is particularly dramatic for those who undergo a surgical menopause—that is, when both ovaries are removed, usually along with the uterus, in a procedure called an oophorectomy. Whereas most women have a good three-to-ten-year period of gradual loss of hormonal production, those who lose their ovaries overnight are jeopardized immediately.

But it is possible to keep all the benefits of estrogen even after menopause, if you replace the hormone pharmaceutically in the body. And in fact most studies show that replacement estrogen really does make a difference in lowering your risk of coronary heart disease. In eleven out of twenty-four published reports, women using unopposed estrogen (without a progestin) had a

50 percent reduction in risk, independent of other risk factors for coronary heart disease.

Taking replacement hormones is not without its drawbacks, however. Medical science has been struggling for a long time now to come up with a medication that will retain the benefits of natural hormonal production after midlife without any detrimental side effects. The quest for the perfect replacement is still ongoing—and we are nowhere near a panacea that's right for every woman—but there have been great advances in both safety and effectiveness over the last twenty-five years.

The History of ERT and HRT (Estrogen Replacement Therapy and Hormone Replacement Therapy)

In the early 1970s, a physician named Robert Wilson discovered that by replacing estrogen in the female body after menopause, he could keep women from undergoing some of the problems associated with menopause. Women bought his book, *Feminine Forever,* and followed his principles, and were thrilled to discover that they were spared the vaginal dryness and hot flashes of their unmedicated sisters. Unfortunately, Dr. Wilson had missed some vital points about replacing hormones. In his regimen, known as ERT (estrogen replacement therapy), he prescribed a very high dosage of estrogen and neglected to pair this hormone with its counterpart, progesterone. Also, he was remiss in monitoring his patients' progress. Because there was no progestin to induce the endometrium (uterine lining) to slough off, overgrowth of the tissue occurred. And so, one year after starting his treatment, women were appearing in doctors' offices with uterine cancer.

Other researchers who came after the disgraced Dr. Wilson made some big changes, so that hormone replacement therapy (HRT) would in fact mimic exactly what the body does when it is cycling naturally. The dosage of estrogen was cut drastically, progesterone was added to the regimen halfway through the month, and women took no pills at all for the final five days, during which time the lining of their uterus was shed in a process that resembled a natural menstrual period.

ERT and HRT—What's the Difference to My Heart?

There are two methods of receiving replacement hormones, ERT (just estrogen) and HRT (estrogen plus a progestin). If you have not had a hysterectomy and still have an intact uterus and uterine lining (the endometrium), you will most likely take HRT. There are certain physicians who will allow a woman with a uterus to take a progestin every *other* month to gain the most cardiovascular benefit from the therapy. However, only monthly use of the progestin can ensure that the lining will not overgrow under the influence of estrogen. But if you have no uterus—and no lining—you may take ERT, without the progestin.

Unfortunately, in terms of the effect on the heart, there's quite a difference. Estrogen is the protective hormone that raises our HDLs and keeps our LDLs and triglycerides at bay. But the synthetic hormone progestin, traditionally prescribed instead of natural progesterone because it is easier to manufacture and is therefore more available, removes some of the excellent benefits.

As mentioned above, if you want to mimic the body's ebb and flow of ovarian hormones and allow the lining of the uterus to slough off every month, you must receive progesterone as well as estrogen.

But progestins tend to raise the LDL level and lower the HDL. They also take away some of the good antioxidant benefits that estrogens have conveyed. (Interestingly enough, so does testosterone, which might be another factor responsible for men having heart attacks at earlier ages.)

But how much less benefit do you get if you add the progestin? It is not exactly clear. Some studies show that a *combined continuous* regimen, where both pills are taken every day without a break, is better for lipid profiles than the *cyclical* method, where the progestin is added for the second half of the cycle. Other studies show that the particular type of progestin may make a difference in keeping HDLs high and LDLs low. A year-long trial showed that women taking .625 milligrams of conjugated estrogen and 2.5 milligrams of medroxyprogesterone acetate maintained HDL levels just as favorable as ones obtained through estrogen use alone.

But adding a progestin makes for certain hormonal discomforts that not every woman will tolerate. If you recall the days of your menstrual cycle, you probably got moody and depressed right before you bled. You might have felt bloated and nauseated, your breasts were sore, and by retaining fluid, you put on water weight. This is exactly what happens to many women during the progestin portion of the HRT regimen.

But there may be new hope for those on the combination therapy. The most recent data, released in November, 1994, from a three-year study of nearly 900 women and funded by the National Institutes of Health, holds out some very interesting possibilities for the future of HRT. This study, called the Post-menopausal Estrogen and Progestin Interventions Trial (PEPI), tested *natural*, or *micronized progesterone* as well as synthetic progestin. The findings were that this form of progesterone caused fewer side effects and was easier to tolerate. It lowered LDLs and raised HDLs better than the progestin, although neither kept HDLs as high as estrogen alone.

Micronized progesterone, made from finely ground soybeans, is only available from certain pharmacies in the United States, and to get an appropriately effective response, the dosage must be considerably larger than that of the synthetic progestin. But in the future, it's certainly possible that micronized progesterone will solve some of the problems that have plagued women who decide to take hormone replacement therapy.

Of course, if you have had a hysterectomy, and don't have a uterus, you don't have to worry about shedding the lining each month. That means you don't need to take a progestin and can gain all the benefits of the therapy with few drawbacks. But can women who still have a uterus get the good cardiovascular effect of replacement estrogen?

The Benefits of HRT

The answer to that question is a qualified yes. We are already aware of the importance of estrogen to our HDLs. Even with a progestin added, we can boost our "good" cholesterol by taking HRT. Additional benefits to replacement estrogen plus progesterone include decreased blood pressure, a more stable environment within the blood vessel (which means less chance of plaques rupturing—the cause of most heart attacks), and improved insulin levels.

Estrogen does a number of other good things that have nothing to do with your lipid profiles. It seems to have a directly protective effect on the arterial wall, preventing it from having spasms and developing lesions. It also allows for good vascular elasticity, permitting the walls to expand and contract under different pressures of blood flow. Another benefit of estrogen is that it seems to reduce the tendency for the body to increase its fat stores—a common phenomenon of aging. Estrogen also acts as an antioxidant—similar to vitamins C, E, and beta-carotene. This means that it may prevent LDLs from being oxidized in the blood and getting into the arterial wall.

Of course, since heart disease is the number-one killer in this country, it is crucial to note that taking HRT can change your risk of dying of cardiovascular disease. Many studies confirm that HRT users reduce their risk of death from coronary vascular disease dramatically—one study in Rochester, Minnesota, found that if all eligible women used HRT, heart attacks could be reduced by 45 percent—about as big a lifesaver as if the women had stopped smoking. The Nurses' Health Study, which recently had its ten-year follow-up, showed the risk of CVD reduced by 50 percent in current users of HRT.

The newest data from the PEPI study mentioned above, however, indicates that a combination of estrogen and progesterone is better than estrogen alone, not only as protection against uterine cancer, but also against heart attacks.

Other studies are not as conclusive, and in many the percentages are considerably smaller, yet the general feeling in the medical establishment is that the longer a woman remains on the therapy, the better her chances of protecting herself from heart disease. The difficult corollary to this is that very few studies span more than ten years (the Women's Health Initiative of the NIH is currently in the midst of a fourteen-year study), and we simply don't know the consequences of therapy beyond that point.

If we look beyond heart disease to other benefits of this therapy, we can find other good reasons for taking HRT. It is a boon for those who are sleepless from hot flashes and sexless from a dry vagina, but the real meaning of replacing hormones in postmenopausal women is in the long-term benefits it can offer our bones.

HRT Reduces the Risk of Osteoporosis

Osteoporosis, which means "porous bones," is known as the silent killer because there are generally no symptoms until the disease is well under way, and it can be deadly. Women, who have lighter, smaller bones than men to begin with, grow increasingly fragile with age when their estrogen supply is no longer sufficient to help retain calcium in the bone tissue. As our supplies of estrogen decrease after menopause, bone mass and density drop radically, and we are increasingly at risk for this painful condition. The multiple vertebral fractures of osteoporosis can leave a woman bent double from "dowager's hump," and a hip fracture can leave her crippled for life or at risk of dying of pneumonia or other complications after surgery.

Numerous studies have shown that HRT significantly improved bone mass and density in postmenopausal women, since estrogen promotes the retention of calcium in bone tissue. This means that you will be less likely to sustain fractures and will retain the enormously important ability to exercise—which of course is essential for good heart health. And if you should happen to have open heart surgery, having good bones is a real bonus. If the sternum and ribs are in good condition, they can be manipulated, cut, and stitched. Poor bone quality would result in poor healing, which could necessitate a surgical repair and would complicate your recovery.

What Are the Drawbacks of HRT?

The issue of breast cancer comes up time and again whenever HRT is discussed. How can we justify handling one disease by predisposing ourselves to another? Some studies indicate that there may be an increased risk of breast cancer in some women on HRT. But it is still unclear as to whether the culprit is a high dosage of estrogen, or the progestin component. The studies that made women so wary about possible breast cancers were performed in Sweden, where the particular types of estrogen and progesterone delivered were substantially different from the types we use in America.

The other cancer that's been associated with HRT is uterine or endometrial cancer. All women who have a uterus must protect the lining from overgrowth—it has to slough off once a month or it can develop cancerous cells. Taking a progestin is the only recourse to keeping a healthy endometrium—even though it does detract from the excellent benefits that estrogen has to impart.

Other risks of taking long-term HRT range from liver and kidney disease to gallstones, to elevated blood pressure, varicose veins and thromboembolic problems.

How Is HRT Administered?

There are several regimens for both ERT and HRT.

1. Oral, Cyclical. Estrogen is given for the first twenty-five days of what will become your "cycle." A progestin is added for days twelve to twenty-five if you have a uterus. You take no supplements for the remainder of the month and then have a "period."

2. Oral, Continuous. Estrogen and progestin are given

daily for those on HRT; estrogen alone for those on ERT. After the first three months, although you may see some spotting, you should have no breakthrough bleeding.

One drawback of oral administration of HRT or ERT is that anything you ingest has to be processed by your liver. There have been instances of liver and gallbladder disease and gall-stones (caused by an increase in bile production in the liver) associated with oral estrogens. Oral estrogens also tend to raise triglyceride levels—and we know that these lipids present an independent risk factor for heart disease in women.

3. Transdermal Patch. A patch with an estrogen reservoir is applied to the hip or buttock and changed twice a week. (An oral progestin is added for those on HRT.) The skin is the semipermeable membrane through which the estrogen enters the body. Most physicians feel that its affect on lipids is as effective as the oral administration, but it takes much longer to see the benefits on a heart with significantly clogged arteries. The patch has its own good points—it bypasses the liver, doesn't raise triglycerides as the pill does, and is particularly helpful to your bones.

4. Percutaneous Gel. This estrogen gel dries into a patch. Same administration as for number 3, above.

5. Subcutaneous Implant. A small estrogen pellet is implanted in the lower abdomen and can be left there for three to six months before it is changed. Some experimental studies have used a Progestasert IUD for the progestin portion of the regimen for those on HRT; others use an oral progestin.

6. Estrogen Cream (for those with or without a uterus, this can be used without a progestin). This topical cream is beneficial for those who only want relief of vaginal dryness. Since it is only used in a localized area two times a week in small amounts, it doesn't do anything to protect the heart. A tiny amount of estrogen passes through the vagina into the bloodstream, but the risk of endometrial thickening is minimal. However, daily use will give the same blood levels of estrogen as the oral regimen.

7. Estrogen in Combination with Other Drugs (for

those with a uterus, these must also be used with a progestin). **Estratest** is a combination of estrogen and testosterone, a gonadal hormone that keeps our libido active. Some women experience an acute drop in production of testosterone after menopause, but luckily, it can be supplemented. The dosage must be carefully measured—trial and error is the key here—so that a woman does feel desire, but not so much that she can't think about anything else.

Estrogen plus an **Antidepressant** are used for women who remain depressed, even under the mood-elevating influence of estrogen alone. You should certainly get a second opinion from a psychotherapist if you feel constantly sad or anxious. Therapy may be of value in addition to or instead of the antidepressant.

Dosage

The lower the dosage, the lower the risk. The most common dosages in the oral regimen are .625 milligrams Premarin and 5 milligrams Provera daily (those with no uterus only take the Premarin). The most common dosage for the patch is either .05 or .1 milligram of estradiol 17-beta. The statistics on increased risk of breast cancer are only significant in amounts of estrogen above .625. Some conservative physicians will start you off on .3 milligrams, but unfortunately, this very low dosage is not sufficient to effect lipid changes or protect the bones, and most women don't see a real difference in hot flashes or vaginal dryness at this level either.

	HRT (estrogen plus progestin)	ERT (estrogen alone)

Benefits	raises HDLs
	good vessel elasticity
	protects bones
	reduces hot flashes
	reduces vaginal dryness and
	  other menopausal
	  symptoms
		raises HDLs
		lowers LDLs
		lowers triglycerides (plus other
		  benefits of HRT)

	HRT (estrogen plus progestin)	ERT (estrogen alone)
Drawbacks	raises LDLs raises triglycerides	
Side Effects	increases risk of endometrial cancer may increase risk of breast cancer kidney/liver disease gallstones thromboembolic problems weight gain fluid retention migraines may raise blood pressure mood swings/depression	increased risk of breast cancer but no risk of endometrial cancer without intact uterus and endometrium (same side effects as HRT but less fluid retention and no mood swings/depression)

Administration	oral
	   cyclic
	     combined continuous
	transdermal patch
	percutaneous gel
	subcutaneous implant
	estrogen cream (all methods must add a progestin except topical cream)
		oral
		   continuous (same administration as HRT but no progestin needed)

Dosages	Oral estrogen (dosages range from .3 to .625 mg. to 1.25 mg. daily) Oral progestin (2.5 to 5 mg. daily) Patch .05 or .1 estradiol 17-beta	oral estrogen or patch same as HRT (no progestin needed)
Other drugs in combination	Estratest (combined estrogen and testosterone) must be given with a progestin HRT plus antidepressant	Estratest (no progestin) ERT plus antidepressant (no progestin needed)
Price	$130 to $150 yearly for estrogen $180 to $210 yearly for progestin	$130 to $150 yearly

Are ERT or HRT Right for Every Postmenopausal Woman?

This is a difficult question and there's a great deal of controversy around the answer.

If you have a history of heart disease in your family and are an otherwise healthy postmenopausal woman, most physicians would give you an emphatic yes, and a "no question about it" if you've had a hysterectomy. The same answer would probably be given to healthy women with no history of heart disease or of cancer of any sort despite the fact that researchers are still unsure as to the safety of taking this medication for longer than ten years, since there are few large-scale studies that go out this far. The answer is a simple no if you have had or currently have an estrogen-dependent cancer. If you took HRT or ERT, you would be endangering your health by increasing the amount of estrogen in your body. No one could justify a treatment that would protect your heart at the risk of your life. A woman with fibrocystic breasts, however, where the lumps are benign and not estrogen dependent, may be a good candidate for replacement as long as she's monitored carefully.

There are other physicians who feel that if you've had any kind of clotting problem, such as stroke, embolism, or deep vein thrombosis, then you shouldn't be on HRT. However, the dosages at which estrogen is delivered in this regimen are low enough so that they usually don't affect the clotting mechanism. But can you trust what's "usual"? You may be the exception to the rule. Prescribing HRT for women with clotting problems is a hard call for many doctors and patients.

Kidney or liver disease and gallstones are three contraindications to taking HRT in its oral form, and sickle-cell anemia is another. But if you have a strong family history of heart disease and your physician is determined to give you the maximum amount of protection, you will probably be advised to wear the transdermal patch (see above)—and of course be monitored carefully.

If you still have a uterus and must take a progestin so that your lining will shed each month, you may feel subject to the enormous emotional changes that are triggered by this hormone. Women who have a tendency to become depressed often feel so "down" during the second half of their cycle when they're under the influence of the progestin that they discontinue the medication entirely. This situation should be discussed with your physician—it is possible that you would benefit from a different dosage, or a combination of estrogen and an antidepressant.

Should You Take Hormones If You Have Diagnosed Heart Disease?

Some physicians feel that the woman who's already had a heart attack or has been diagnosed with coronary artery disease is the best candidate for estrogen replacement, at least on a short-term basis. If you are already in the group designated the most likely to die from cardiovascular disease, and you can improve your lipid profile with estrogen, you probably stand a good chance of living longer on HRT or ERT.

Unfortunately, there have been few studies exclusively dedicated to looking at the long-term benefits for those with preexisting coronary heart disease. Currently, a five-year trial—the HERS study (Heart and Estrogen-progestin Replacement Study)—is being conducted in fifteen centers to investigate the effects of hormone replacement on non-hysterectomized postmenopausal women with heart disease. The results, which will be available in 1998, will give more of us the opportunity to make an informed choice about this therapy.

There are types of heart disease, however, that make HRT inadvisable. If you've suffered a pulmonary embolism or deep vein thrombosis, this treatment is not for you. The possibility of activating another blood clot would be too dangerous.

What about other heart disorders? Women with coronary artery stenosis have been shown to improve their outcomes with hormone replacement. The improvement of HDL and LDL levels are certainly important, but perhaps what's more significant in this cardiac condition is the effect estrogen has on the elasticity of the blood vessel walls.

How to Work with Your Physician to Make an HRT Decision

After the most obvious drawbacks and side effects have been factored out, the answer to the question becomes hazier. Should every woman who no longer menstruates be on a medication for thirty or forty years to replace a hormone that she has stopped producing naturally? Should a healthy person be medicated for a condition she may never get?

How do you decide and which doctor do you consult in order to make this decision?

Your cardiologist prescribes only drugs that affect the heart directly; your gynecologist or family practitioner is the person to see if you are considering HRT or ERT and your cardiologist thinks it would be advisable for you to protect your heart with hormones. But you must understand that the two of them may have a difference of opinion when it comes to how to administer the regimen and what should be included in your "mix."

If you still have a uterus, the gynecologist will probably suggest that you take either the cyclic or the combined continuous oral dosage—that is, two pills, one of estrogen and one of a progestin. You would take the continuous dosage of estrogen only if you have no uterus.

The cardiologist would undoubtedly prefer that you take no progestin, *even if you have a uterus,* and here the conflict of interests becomes more difficult. As was mentioned earlier, there are gynecologists who will allow you to skip the progestin every other month and some will actually permit you to go three months without it as long as they monitor the endometrium with a vaginal ultrasound or an endometrial biopsy every three to six months. But the biopsy is invasive and uncomfortable and both procedures are costly—not to mention anxiety provoking and possibly risky.

The dosage of your estrogen is another vital factor. You will recall that women on birth control pills—particularly those who smoke—are at high risk for clotting problems, such as stroke or embolism. The amount of estrogen in a birth control pill is much higher than the standard dosage of .625 milligrams of estrogen in an HRT or ERT regimen. It would be risky for a woman who has already had a heart attack to be placed on a regimen with a higher estrogen dosage just to get a better effect on her lipid profile. Your gynecologist must be aware of these dangers for a woman with heart disease.

So some difficult choices hang in the balance for you and your two physicians.

How do you decide? Clearly, you are not a trained professional, and you must listen to the physicians you've consulted. If they disagree, they will undoubtedly talk to each other and come up with a compromise that's suitable to all parties.

But you must not allow others to make this choice for you. If you are a very high risk candidate for heart disease, and you have had a hysterectomy, the decision is clear—you should be taking estrogen if you have never had an estrogen-dependent cancer.

If you still have a uterus, but you are high risk for heart disease, the data suggests that you will live longer and better on HRT. If you are a low-risk candidate for heart disease but a high risk for one or several types of cancer, you may opt not to start this regimen. As it happens, only 20 percent of postmenopausal women in this country ever start HRT and only 10 percent continue past the first year. The lack of compliance shows how nervous we all are about taking a medication for a life condition—no one ever told our grandmothers they should take a drug when they were healthy in order to live longer.

To start thinking seriously about this choice, make yourself a list of pros and cons and then weigh the outcomes with your medical professional. We must examine the positives and negatives, and we can only do this if we look at our whole health picture objectively. Here's a comparison, for those who are considering HRT.

Positives for HRT

- improves lipid profile

- improves vascular elasticity

- more beta-endorphins
  (improves mood)
- reduces vaginal dryness
  (improves sexual response,
  which may improve mood)
- reduces hot flashes (fewer stress
  hormones produced)
- improves bone density and
  mass

Negatives Against HRT

- increases risk of breast and
  endometrial cancer
- may induce clotting or
  thrombosis and bring on stroke
- may predispose you to
  gallstones
- may predispose you to kidney
  and liver disease

- may elevate blood pressure

- may exacerbate varicose veins

- progestin portion of regimen
  may give you the "blues"

HRT or ERT will not change your whole health picture. You must obviously be attentive to all the other preventive-care tactics we've outlined earlier. Remember too that no decision is irrevocable. What you and your physician think is right for you today may change in five or ten years. And as the field grows and medical research becomes more sophisticated, the answers for which we're searching may become clearer. Until then, we have only our own good consciences—and our hearts—to guide us.

7

When Something Goes Wrong: Problems in and Around the Heart

∇

The heart, as we've learned, is an enormously complex organ, and everything in the body depends on it functioning properly. Not only do we have to rely on a healthy heart, we also need to know that the entire circulatory system is in good shape. Unfortunately, when one element is out of alignment, other elements follow suit.

Heart disease covers the gamut—from coronary artery disease to congenital defects to the mysterious Syndrome X (which affects mostly women) to hypertension to arrhythmias to sudden death. You not only have to understand your symptoms but also be absolutely clear when you present them to your health-care professional so as not to have the same awful experience Grace did.

At thirty-four, Grace was a small, lithe black woman, weighing barely 115 pounds. Married, with four children, managing a difficult career, she never expected to get sick. As an oncology nurse at a local hospital, she had her cholesterol checked once a year at her annual physical. She never smoked, ate a healthy diet, and was very physically active. How could she have a heart attack? She never gave a thought to her family legacy of heart disease, which in cases such as hers, overrides both general good health and the premenopausal protection of estrogen.

Two weeks before the event, Grace started feeling some pain under her sternum in the center of her chest. It would move up and radiate out to her left arm. She figured it was indigestion, took some Maalox and Mylanta, and the pain went away. But it came back, and kept coming back, for four days.

On the fifth day, she drove to the emergency room with acute pain, nauseated, with bouts of feeling feverish and then chilled. "They did an ECG and an X ray, and they were both negative. The doctor thought I had maybe a flu or a virus, so he sent me home, told me to keep taking the Mylanta.

"I barely functioned during the week, but Friday, I went to my son's football game. We were in the bleachers when the pain got worse and moved down to my left arm and leg. I felt numb along the left side of my body. I was cold and clammy and nauseated again.

"My husband carried me to the van and drove to the emergency room. The same doctors were there from the week before, and they did the same two tests, and they told me the same thing—everything normal. This time they gave me the name of a gastroenterologist.

"The weekend was awful—I couldn't even lie flat in the bed because I was in so much pain. So Monday, I went to see the GI specialist and he did an ECG in the office. Nothing. He told me he thought I had an ulcer or a hernia, and he put me on Zantac and ordered a GI series two weeks from that day.

"By Friday, I was in the worst pain of my life. I said to myself, This is a heart attack. It was nearly impossible for me to get to the phone and call my husband, and as soon as I did, I passed out on the floor. He got me to the emergency room, and this time, we weren't leaving. I asked to be admitted. They did another ECG and wanted to discharge me. I was getting hysterical and asked for a nitroglycerin. I figured, if it was a heart attack, it would help, and if it wasn't, it wouldn't hurt.

"This emergency room doctor I'd now seen three times refused to give me the medication until I said, 'I have insurance, they'll pay,' and he finally gave it to me to pacify me. But the pain was gone in about fifteen seconds, so I kept thinking I had to be right.

"My husband refused to sign the discharge slip and we went over this guy's head to get me admitted. But it wasn't until Saturday night that the weekend cardiologist on duty came in to read the new ECG's and asked, 'Where's the thirty-four-year-old with the massive heart attack?' "

Grace was transferred from this local hospital to a nearby medical center for an emergency catheterization. During the procedure, they dissected her main artery by accident and had to perform an emergency double bypass. She "died" twice on the table and had to be revived with the defibrillator.

Grace was hospitalized for three months. She lay in a comalike state for weeks, the front wall of her heart permanently damaged, compounded by mitral valve regurgitation. When she was finally discharged the day before Christmas, 1991, she had to learn to walk all over again. She was weak, short of breath, totally reliant on medication.

Why didn't Grace get the care she needed? Why would no one believe this young, healthy woman was having a heart attack? The most likely possibility is that she suffered a spasm in her artery, but it was intermittent and didn't happen each time she had an ECG. The final reading that the cardiologists did, however, showed that her T-waves were inverted—clearly a cardiac abnormality. (See Chapter 8 for an explanation of how an ECG is read.)

The multiple mistakes that led to Grace's horrendous experience didn't have to happen. If the emergency room doctors had called in a cardiologist for a consult, if she had had a proper workup when her chest pains got intense, if the GI man had decided that her problem had nothing to do with his specialty, she might have been cared for sooner and better. But the most glaring error, according to Grace, was her own lack of perseverance. "I was too passive. I just got hysterical and they didn't believe me. I should have stuck to my guns and just stayed there the first time and demanded to see a doctor who could figure out what was wrong with me. You have to be your own advocate in the health-care system—because nobody else will do it for you."

The Symptoms of Women's Heart Disease

In your heart of hearts, you know when you're sick and you know when you're well. But many women ignore the symptoms of heart disease for years, and in so doing, are able to con themselves into believing that something "abnormal" is perfectly normal.

The following symptoms are *not* normal, and should be taken seriously. If you experience any of these regularly, you should see your physician and be perfectly honest when she asks for occasions and intensity of the experience:

1. chest pain (particularly centered)
2. palpitations (pounding of the heart), bumping, fluttering, or flopping
3. blackouts or fainting
4. shortness of breath
5. great fatigue

CHEST PAIN

Angina is the typical primary warning sign of heart disease. But angina resembles other types of pain as well. Women often have heart rhythm disturbances and chest pain caused by hiatal hernias, gallbladder disease, or anxiety.

As described in *The Mayo Clinic Heart Book,* the pain of angina can be:

crushing	squeezing
constricting	burning
aching	strangling

pressure	like a gas pain
heavy	full
tight	like indigestion
cold	choking
clammy	makes you weak

Angina generally appears when you're exerting yourself—climbing, hammering, shoveling snow, feeling emotionally overwhelmed. It comes on as a tightness in the chest and may radiate out to the jaw and left arm and shoulder blade (although sometimes it may also move to the right arm). It increases in intensity until it hits its peak, which generally causes the individual to sit down and rest, at which point it vanishes. The reason is that when you're under pressure or moving quickly, the heart needs but isn't receiving enough oxygen because the arteries are too narrow to allow continuous blood flow. When you rest, of course, the heart doesn't need as much oxygen. **Stable angina** is angina that has been predictably present for some time, that is, the patient can predict which activities will provoke it. This type of angina also responds to nitroglycerin tablets under the tongue.

Unstable angina may appear at any time and may fluctuate in intensity. The individual starts having these episodes more frequently, and it doesn't take much effort to bring them on. The pain may persist or occur even when you sit or lie down to rest.

The pain of **variant** or **vasospastic** angina may awaken you from a deep sleep in the middle of the night—it doesn't take any exertion to bring it on. It may last for up to half an hour, and reaches its peak quickly. This is also called **Prinzmetal's** angina. Typical sufferers are younger individuals who are heavy smokers. This type of pain is not caused by blockage in the major arteries but rather by a spasm in a blood vessel as it expands and contracts. This was probably the type of extreme pain experienced by Grace. It never showed up on any of her numerous ECGs because she wasn't spasming at the time of her tests.

PALPITATIONS

When you are anxious or eager to see someone or experiencing stage fright, you heart will begin to pound. The body is able to cope with changes in the pumping mechanism—as long as it doesn't vacillate for protracted periods of time.

But true palpitations are caused by **arrhythmias,** or irregular heartbeats. The feeling of pounding or bumping is usually accompanied by pain and may make it very difficult for you to breathe. Unlike the swoony "missed beat" you feel when you encounter a loved one, palpitations may go on for hours. This is a clear indication that the regular rhythm of the heart is disturbed. (See below for a discussion of arrhythmias.)

BLACKOUTS

Blackouts are terrifying events, not only for the person experiencing the episode but also for witnesses. And if you're behind the wheel of a car when it happens, this can be a potentially fatal symptom.

If you are a person who typically feels faint during circumstances as varied as being in a crowded elevator, taking a hot bath, getting up too quickly after a big meal, or when you're dehydrated and keep on exercising, you are probably just a victim of **orthostatic hypotension,** a situation where the blood pressure falls rapidly, or **vasovagal syncope,** which is caused by overstimulation of the vagus nerve, which helps to regulate breathing and circulation.

However, if you find that you are having blackouts on a regular basis, without any warning—no nausea, dizziness, or lightheadedness before you faint—you may have a cardiac problem. Arrhythmias and valve defects both cause this type of instantaneous blackout.

SHORTNESS OF BREATH

You may not have the same get-up-and-go that you had thirty years ago, but it is the rare fifty-year-old who can keep up in a race with her eight-year-old grandson. Some shortness of breath naturally comes with age, since we gradually lose lung capacity (unless we're marathon swimmers or runners) after midlife.

However, if you are severely winded after climbing a flight of stairs, you may have a cardiac problem. If you awake from sleep with a feeling that you can't get a complete breath, and even raising yourself up on pillows doesn't help, you may be experiencing heart failure.

Being out of shape and overweight can make it harder for you to breathe. But this significant symptom should not be overlooked if you are concerned about your heart health.

SWELLING OF BODY PARTS

The puffy look of many individuals with heart disease is caused by **edema,** a condition where the body retains water. A typical symptom of heart failure is **pitting edema,** where you can press into the skin of the leg and leave a depression. The water retained in the body accumulates in the tissues. Edema associated with heart disease is most commonly seen in the ankles and lower legs, where the fluid pools because of gravity.

FATIGUE

This is a particularly hard one for doctors to deal with. Any woman who comes into a physician's office complaining of just this one symptom will undoubtedly be patted on the back and told to "take it easy."

You should first evaluate other reasons for feeling tired, such as working extra hard, being depressed, not eating or sleeping well because of anxiety, or because you've recently been ill and are just recovering.

The type of fatigue associated with heart disease is usually overwhelming and distinctly out of pattern. It is a fatigue that makes you feel very different from your usual self. If you are generally a person who gets up with the sun and walks a brisk two miles each morning and you suddenly find that you cannot drag yourself out of bed, or you're exhausted after climbing a flight of stairs, this might be a symptom of heart disease.

If You've Got Symptoms, What's Wrong with Your Heart?

The confusing thing about all the symptoms mentioned above is that many of them could apply to several different types of heart disease, and for that matter, to many other illnesses that have nothing to do with your heart.

It takes teamwork on the part of patient and physician to put the pieces of this puzzle together. This is why you must learn to express yourself in very accurate terms and make sure by asking questions that you've been heard and understood. Everything you tell the doctor—family history, lifestyle, risk factors, other physical or mental conditions, medications you currently take, recent traumas you've experienced, *as well as* the symptoms mentioned above will be brush strokes that eventually come together to create a full portrait of your illness.

The types of heart problems are many and varied. The most common, which we'll discuss in this chapter, are:

- coronary artery disease
- silent ischemia
- Syndrome X
- stroke
- cardiac arrhythmias
- hypertensive cardiovascular disease
- pulmonary hypertension
- congenital heart defects
  stenosis: aortic and pulmonary
  septal defects: atrial and ventricular
- mitral valve prolapse
- pericarditis
- congestive heart failure
- sudden death

Coronary Artery Disease

The most common form of heart disease for males and females in this country is coronary artery disease. This disease is also the one responsible for most heart attacks. If the arteries that permit blood flow to the heart are blocked for as little as half an hour, the heart itself can suffer permanent damage from its lack of oxygen, and this may result in disability or even death.

The interior of each artery is initially a hollow, expansive tube. But as years pass, various waste products collect inside these passageways. Fatty deposits known as plaque are the worst offenders, and these settle in on the interior of the vessels. This condition is called **atherosclerosis.**

The greater the blockage, the narrower the passageway available to carry the blood supply. As the inside of the arteries hardens with plaque, it becomes increasingly difficult for the heart to receive the blood supply it needs. This condition, known as **ischemia,** may not result in permanent damage to the myocardium. How dangerous the ischemia can become depends on the size of the artery that's blocked and whether the blockage—or **occlusion**—is gradual or sudden, complete or incomplete. When a plaque completely blocks an artery leading to the heart, it can cause a heart attack. If there's an occlusion in an artery that leads to the brain, it can cause a stroke; elsewhere in the body, a blockage can cause poor circulation to the legs or kidney damage. Atherosclerosis does *not* form blood clots—actually what happens is that in the arteries, blood clots form as a consequence of the rupture of an atherosclerotic plaque.

Atheromas or **atheromatous plaques** start forming in childhood if we eat poorly and don't exercise enough, and they get progressively worse over the years. The long, slow process of atherosclerosis can take twenty years or more—however, the good news is that we can stop or even reverse these blockages with careful attention to preventive care (see Chapters 4, 5, and 6).

But how did those blockages get there in the first place? This is not clearly understood because there are so many factors at work. Let's look at the degenerative changes that go on inside the artery as well.

The lining of the wall, called the **endothelium,** can sustain just so much injury from elevation of blood pressure and stresses on the arterial wall. As these walls get thicker and less elastic over the years from free-radical damage, they also become roughened. Chemical and mechanical pressures break down the barrier between the cells that line the arteries and allow fat cells to get underneath and remain there. (The job of antioxidants is to protect against or reduce this type of damage, which is why a balanced diet including vitamin and mineral supplementation is the very basis of a healthy heart program. See Chapter 4 for a listing of antioxidants.)

The body reacts to this damage to arterial walls with a proliferation of smooth muscle cells, which in combination with the fatty deposits allow microscopic blood clots to form on the surface of the artery wall. Over time, as this collection of clots and fat matures, it becomes an atherosclerotic plaque.

The plaque is not a rigid element, however. It has dynamic movement, and as it gets larger, it is more volatile. Eventually, the plaque can rupture like a volcano, and the body's response is to form a blood clot or **thrombus** on top of it. This thrombus can entirely occlude a blood vessel, cutting off the blood supply and causing a heart attack, also known as an **infarction.**

Was it the elevation of cholesterol in the body that allowed those fat cells to be deposited? Or was it the damage to the endothelium that occurred from the rise in blood pressure? Which came first? Since we don't know, we must try to prevent both from happening—we must keep cholesterol and blood pressure low, and lower or reduce all the other risks that might create damage to the arteries (see Chapter 3).

Symptoms. Angina, palpitations, shortness of breath, great fatigue, heart attacks.

Treatment. Diet and exercise modification, medication, (beta-blockers, calcium channel blockers, nitrates, aspirin, cholesterol-lowering drugs). If these fail, then balloon angioplasty (PTCA) or bypass surgery (CABG).

Silent Ischemia

If you never have pain, you may never know that your heart has been deprived of as much oxygen in an attack of silent ischemia as it might be in an attack of angina. This condition may show up on an ECG or stress test. Sometimes, patients are monitored for twenty-four hours on a Holter monitor (see Chapter 8)—but this test would be performed only if your physician suspected that you might have heart disease. Silent ischemia is common in diabetics who tend to suffer from different types of neuropathy, an affliction of the nerves that causes sensory disturbances. Very often, the diabetic has lost sensation in the body and doesn't feel pain.

Treatment. Medication (same as for angina, above) can be helpful to improve blood flow, and angioplasty may also be recommended.

Syndrome X

The main symptom of Syndrome X is occasional intense anginal pain. Fully two-thirds of the cases that have been identified occur in women. This illness may be almost exclusively the province of peri- and postmenopausal women because of the rapid drop in estrogen production that affects the small blood vessels. It is particularly prevalent in women who have had surgical menopause—that is, their ovaries have been removed—which stops hormonal production immediately.

Syndrome X is difficult to diagnose because most women who have it have no risk factors for heart disease. They may be otherwise healthy individuals who sometimes experience agonizing anginal pain.

This pain, however, is not caused by a blockage in any major arteries—and indeed, a catheterization and angiogram might read normal—because the problem is microscopic. This trouble with the microregulation of blood supply to the cells is at a level too small to be seen on an X ray.

Remember that the circulation system goes way beyond the heart and its feeder veins and arteries. We also rely on the tiny blood vessels that carry the blood and oxygen from the coronary arteries to the other cells of the heart. Researchers suspect that the abnormalities of the small vessels are different from those of the great vessels—Syndrome X is probably an abnormality of something called "flow-reserve." When a woman is undergoing physical or emotional stress, her distal blood vessels (the smallest blood vessels in the heart) may not be dilating sufficiently—either because of her lack of estrogen or some other factor that hasn't yet been identified.

The great pain associated with this syndrome may be caused by a hypersensitivity of the nerves leading to the heart, esophagus, and chest.

Syndrome X doesn't require surgery, and the traditional heart drugs may alleviate the problem. However, putting a woman on a course of hormone replacement therapy or the antidepressant Elavil may be helpful.

Symptoms. Occasional intense anginal pain.

Treatment. Hormone replacement therapy, Elavil, calcium blockers, and/or nitrates, depending on patient.

Stroke

A stroke is a circulatory event that takes place when blood flow cannot reach the brain. This causes many brain cells to die or be irreparably damaged. The functions those cells control—speech, movement, memory, or vision—are consequently impaired or lost.

Approximately 90,000 women a year die of stroke. A stroke—although it involves the brain—is a cardiovascular disease. If the blood supply to the brain is cut off by an atherosclerotic plaque or a clot that's formed in the brain or traveled there from somewhere else in the body, the following may occur:

Symptoms

* weakness and numbness in the limbs, face, or down one side of the body
* inability to speak clearly or understand what others are saying to you
* sudden impaired vision in one eye
* loss of consciousness
* dizziness or falling

Strokes often accompany other cardiac events—the type of arrhythmia known as atrial fibrillation may disturb the regular pumping action of the heart sufficiently to form a clot, which may travel to the brain. A malfunctioning valve may prohibit the blood from flowing freely through the heart, which may lead to the blood thickening and forming a clot. Even open heart surgery may leave the body susceptible to stroke.

There are several different types of strokes:

Cerebral thrombosis: In the same way that plaque builds up on the walls of coronary arteries, so can it build up on the wall of an artery leading from the heart to the neck or brain. If a clot (thrombosis) develops on the plaque, it blocks blood flow to the brain, and a stroke will result.

Cerebral hemorrhage: This occurs when a blood vessel ruptures in the brain.

Cerebral embolism: A blood clot forms elsewhere in the body (usually in the hearts of patients with coronary artery disease or valvular disease) and travels through the bloodstream to an artery feeding the brain, causing a blockage.

Treatment. Physical and speech rehabilitation are the key elements of stroke recovery for those who survive. Graded strength exercises can train limbs to function well again, and detailed memory work and practice on various word drills can assist in the recovery of impaired areas of speech. Occupational therapy can be extremely beneficial—there are all sorts of special tools and devices that can be made for individuals with stroke to ease their passage back to health.

It can be harder to recover well from a stroke than from a heart attack, because each part of the brain is responsible for a specific type of body function. When one area of the brain is damaged, sometimes other areas can take over the function in time. However, extensive damage to the brain may leave permanent impairment or weakness or lead to death.

Rehabilitation is most successful when the patient is motivated to get well. (Lack of motivation, unfortunately, can be one manifestation of this event.) If the damage to the brain has not been too extensive, it is possible to recoup some or all of one's mental and physical capacities.

Cardiac Arrhythmias

Atrial fibrillation and *atrial flutter* are two types of arrhythmias that can be controlled with changes in your lifestyle as well as medication.

Atrial fibrillation occurs when the walls of the upper chambers of the heart (the left and right atria) start to contract in a rapid, nonrhythmic beat. This type of abnormal contraction may be as fast as three hundred irregular beats a minute. This can occur after a heart attack, or to people who have atherosclerosis, rheumatic heart disease, angina, or congestive heart failure. It may be a rare, occasional event, or it can be chronic. If atrial fibrillation continues unchecked, the heart can beat at a very fast rate and cause symptoms of chest pain, dizziness or breathlessness. It can also encourage the development of blood clots that may travel and block the carotid artery and cause a stroke.

If the cells in the lower chambers lose their rhythm, this is *ventricular fibrillation*. This type of arrhythmia stops the ventricles from contracting in an organized way and prevents the blood from flowing out to the rest of the body. If this situation isn't reversed, death will result. Ventricular fibrillation usually occurs when a heart attack is in progress and must be converted with an electric shock.

PAT or *paroxysmal atrial tachycardia,* also known as *atrial flutter,* occurs when the atria contract at a rate that is much faster than normal. The ventricles may respond and will start contracting quickly, creating a fast heartbeat. The tachycardia can be more serious than atrial fibrillation even though it doesn't create an irregular heartbeat. You may be given an electrophysiology (EPS) test (see Chapter 8) to isolate the problem your heart is having with the electrical impulses that are causing the arrhythmias.

Heart block occurs when there is a failure in the passage of electrical impulses through the heart. This usually occurs in patients over sixty-five and may cause dizziness, fainting, or may bring on a stroke. An overdose of Digoxin can trigger a heart block, but so can other medications, hypertension, or coronary artery disease.

Treatment. Antiarrhythmia medications of several varieties are prescribed (see Chapter 9 for the particular types) and must be titrated precisely for each individual patient. You should also avoid caffeine, salt, alcohol, and of course eliminate smoking from your life. In some cases, cardioversion is performed with a machine that shocks the heart and changes the electrical impulse.

If slow heart rhythms are your problem, your doctor may advise that you have an *artificial pacemaker* installed. This small, battery-operated device has saved many lives by taking over the job of producing electrical impulses for the heart. Pacemakers are surgically implanted in a pocket that is created under the skin on the chest, and two leads are inserted into the heart through a vein.

Every pacemaker is individually programmed to suit the particular heart it is helping. Some work around the clock, others only work on demand—when a heart slows below a certain preset rate.

A newer version of a pacemaker known as an *automatic implantable cardioverter defibrillator (AICD)* acts like a traditional exterior defibrillator with paddles—except this one is small enough to implant in the abdominal cavity. The AICD goes into action whenever an arrhythmia occurs, shocking the heart back into a normal rhythm.

Another solution to some arrhythmias is *catheter ablation,* in which radio-frequency energy is delivered via catheter to the affected portion of the heart that malfunctions. This permanently cures the arrhythmia.

Hypertensive Cardiovascular Disease (Hypertension)

Many people live with high blood pressure and manage it well with diet, exercise, and stress-reduction techniques. But since hypertension is usually symptom free, you may not even know you've been living with high blood pressure for years. If it remains constantly elevated, this can lead to severe cardiac problems.

When your pressure is elevated, this means that blood travels through the arteries against high pressure, and the heart must work harder and uses more oxygen to do its work. It may actually demand more oxygen than the coronary arteries can supply. This high pressure in the arteries can severely damage the arterial walls. Changes on the interior of the walls can make them susceptible to the build-up of plaque, which can develop into atherosclerosis.

If the arteries are narrow and rigid to begin with, they will create resistance to the blood flow. The heart's walls may thicken, and as the heart pumps and presses against the narrowed interior, it may dilate. So one factor plays on another, and eventually heart failure may result.

The best way to avoid this type of heart disease is to work closely with your doctor. If you know what your typical range of blood pressure is and have found that diet and exercise are not keeping it under control, you will be placed on a medication to keep it in check. Even if you feel much better, don't ever stop taking your blood pressure medication without your doctor's okay.

Symptoms. Usually none, or possibly headache or shortness of breath.

Treatment. Preventive care including a low-sodium as well as a low-fat diet, weight loss, exercise, and stress reduction. There is a wide range of various blood-pressure medications that might be prescribed, including ACE inhibitors, calcium blockers, alpha or beta blockers, centrally active agents, and diuretics.

Pulmonary Hypertension

High blood pressure in the lungs is a dangerous type of hypertension that develops in the blood vessels of your respiratory system. Someone with emphysema or chronic pulmonary obstruction may develop this type of hypertension, which can lead to heart failure. A prominent symptom of this disease is a swelling of the body, especially the legs and stomach. This occurs because the increased pressure prevents the right ventricle from pumping blood into the lungs.

Symptoms. Edema, fatigue.

Treatment. There is little that can be done to treat pulmonary hypertension, even if the cause is known. Any treatment would be for the causative illness, such as COPD (chronic obstructive pulmonary disease) or emphysema.

Congenital Heart Defects

A condition is congenital when you are born with it. Congenital heart defects occur when the alignment of structures or formation of tissues doesn't happen at the appropriate time in utero. Sometimes there is one abnormality; sometimes, a cluster. The fetus, using its mother's bloodstream, lungs, and digestive system through its umbilical connection, doesn't need the heart to beat properly until after birth. Initially, the heart is a single tubelike structure that divides into four chambers and develops valves. No one is exactly certain what causes congenital defects—although females are more likely than males to get them.

At least 500,000 Americans live comfortably with some type of congenital heart defect—and many go undiagnosed because they aren't severe enough to impair one's lifestyle. But when the condition begins to inflict damage on the heart, symptoms will appear and must be treated, generally with surgery.

Symptoms

- heart murmur (the doctor can hear the sound of abnormal blood flow)
- palpitations (problems with the electrical system of the heart—this can manifest itself in fainting)
- inability to exercise without exhaustion
- irregularities in blood pressure
- shortness of breath

Defects generally fall into two major categories: either obstruction or rerouting of blood flow. Both of these types of defects make the heart work harder than it should, so that over time it becomes enlarged or weakened.

MALFORMATIONS FROM OBSTRUCTION

Stenosis. These defects result from an *obstruction* of blood flow. The most common stenoses are *pulmonary stenosis* and *aortic stenosis*. (However, any of the four valves may be narrowed or even missing an opening entirely.) The stenosis ("narrowing") that may occur in any of the heart's valves blocks the passage of blood and makes the ventricle work harder than it should.

In pulmonary stenosis, the pulmonary valve, which allows blood to pass from the right ventricle to the lungs, is narrowed. This requires the right ventricle to take the burden of the pumping work, which enlarges the muscle.

Symptoms. Shortness of breath.

Treatment. A procedure similar to angioplasty called balloon valvuloplasty may be used to open the narrowed valve. It can also be surgically widened.

In aortic stenosis, the aortic valve is malformed. This valve, which should have three leaflets, sometimes develops only one or two. These leaflets tend to thicken and block the flow of blood. This means that the ventricle has to work harder to push blood through the narrowed valve.

Symptoms. Usually none until adulthood, then angina, fainting, and heart failure.

Treatment. Balloon valvuloplasty to stretch the valve; valve replacement.

LEFT-TO-RIGHT SHUNT MALFORMATIONS

Some congenital defects such as "holes in the heart" cause a *rerouting* of blood flow. Instead of proceeding normally from right atrium to right ventricle to left atrium to left ventricle (see Chapter 2 for a full explanation of how the heart works), the blood flow takes different paths. A *shunt* causes abnormal entry of blood from one side of the heart to the other. A right-to-left shunt, where venous blood passes into the left atrium or ventricle and then goes out to the rest of the body, results in a "blue baby." A left-to-right shunt results in arterial blood passing into the right side of the heart.

Septal Defects, Atrial and Ventricular (ASD and VSD). Septal defects are holes in the wall that divides the heart in half. This opening in the septum occurs when the two sides of the heart don't close up at birth. These are the most common forms of heart defect.

An *atrial septal defect* means that there is a hole in the wall (or septum) that divides the right and left atria. With a *ventricular septal defect,* there is a hole in the wall that divides the right and left ventricle.

Symptoms. A physician may be able to hear a murmur in an individual with these defects. However, a few cases are not diagnosed until midlife when shortness of breath and arrhythmias become a problem.

Treatment. Surgical correction to mend the opening. Some defects of the atria can be closed without surgery using a catheter technique.

Mitral Valve Prolapse

A seemingly hereditary disorder that tends to run in families, mitral valve prolapse is more common in women than in men and may go undetected for years. About 5 to 7 percent of the general population have this disorder; but 5 to 10 percent of all women have this disorder. It is very often asymptomatic but can be detected during a physical exam. It is more specifically diagnosed by echocardiogram (see Chapter 8). When the mitral valve is prolapsed, it is enlarged and "floppy." That is, instead of snapping neatly closed as blood leaves the left atrium for the ventricle, the leaflets billow out, which allows for leakage in the system. The leaflets bulge upward into the left atrium during ventricular systole, so that blood regurgitates backward into the atrium. In some cases the leaflets prolapse without leaking.

In most types of mitral valve prolapse, a systolic "click" (a snapping sound that occurs near the middle of the ventricular contraction) followed by a murmur (the sound of the blood leaking backward from the valve into the left atrium) will be heard. In other, more severe types, some blood will regurgitate freely back through the valve. If it is very severe, repair or replacement of the valve may be necessary.

In decades past, doctors used to characterize a "typical" MVP patient as a thin, nervous, high-strung woman prone to anxiety attacks. This is evidently a stereotype that must be banished from modern medical thinking—there are plenty of reasonable, heavyset women with this syndrome and many men suffer from it as well. The alleged "nervousness" was often caused by having a sudden onset of symptoms. But when the patient was informed and knew where her symptoms came from, she no longer panicked. However, anxiety and panic attacks do occur in some patients with mitral valve prolapse.

Although there is generally no life-threatening aspect to MVP, it does leave one at greater risk for *bacterial endocarditis,* an infection of the lining of the heart, usually localized to the valves' leaflets. This is why it is so important to take charge of your health and be alert to any situation that might introduce bacteria into your system, for example, undergoing some dental or surgical procedure.

Symptoms. When they do occur, mitral valve symptoms are manifested by chest pain that is quite different from angina. It is usually a brief stabbing pain to the left of the breastbone that occurs at intervals rather than consistently, as with angina. It may be accompanied by palpitations, dizziness, numbness, arrhythmias, fatigue (particularly on exertion), and sometimes neuropsychiatric symptoms such as panic attacks or anxiety.

Symptoms of endocarditis include: high fever and chills, shortness of breath, tachycardia. It may also manifest itself in great fatigue, loss of appetite, night sweats, body ache and headache.

Treatment. All women with MVP should be followed by a physician and have an echocardiogram to confirm the diagnosis, even if they are asymptomatic. They should avoid stimulants such as caffeine, alcohol, and recreational drugs and of course should abstain from smoking. Beta blockers or calcium channel blockers can be useful for those with chest pain, and antibiotics should be given to individuals with a murmur before dental work and certain surgical procedures.

Pericarditis

This syndrome involves an inflammation of the sac that surrounds the heart. It brings with it pain on breathing or a change of posture—particularly when getting into a prone position—and is often accompanied by fever. It is usually triggered by a viral infection, such as a bad case of the flu, and may also occur after a heart attack or as a complication of open heart surgery.

Symptoms. Typical flu symptoms, pain when inhaling or when getting into a prone position.

Treatment. Antiinflammatory drugs are used to bring down the inflammation in the pericardium.

Congestive Heart Failure

In the condition known as congestive heart failure or *cardiac failure*, the heart "fails" to meet the oxygen and metabolic needs of the body. Over three million Americans currently are affected by heart failure, and typically most patients are over sixty-five years of age.

The syndrome sounds dire, and in fact is very often predictive of a shortened life span. The mortality rate is greater than 50 percent at five years no matter what therapy is used. Heart failure is even more serious when complicated by other cardiac problems.

The attempt of all therapy is to strengthen the weakened heart, which isn't pumping enough blood to feed all the various organs and tissues it must supply, and to reduce its workload. Congestive heart failure is often present when there's something else wrong with the heart, such as late-stage severe hypertension, coronary artery disease, heart attack or heart valve malfunctions, which obviously must also be diagnosed and treated.

As heart failure progresses, there may be severe salt and water retention, pulmonary congestion which makes breathing difficult or impossible, or venous system congestion, causing swelling of the legs and abdomen. The work load of the heart increases, but its pumping and contracting abilities decrease. This causes enormous fatigue, because the heart can't keep up with the demands placed on it.

A definitive diagnosis can be made with physical examination, chest X ray, echocardiography or MUGA scanning (see Chapter 8 for an explanation of these tests).

Symptoms
- shortness of breath, especially episodes of being awakened from sleep feeling that you are suffocating
- coughing or wheezing
- swelling caused by water retention, particularly in the legs
- rapid heartbeat
- enormous fatigue

And in extreme cases:

• impaired kidney function
• mental confusion

The heart goes through a variety of mechanisms to compensate for its failure. The first thing that usually happens is that the ventricles enlarge to hold a greater volume of blood. As more blood is held in the chamber, the heart is stretched beyond its limits, which in turn makes for a weaker systolic contraction.

The dilation of the ventricles is an adaptive technique for the heart to be able to pump more blood when it contracts, but unfortunately, in heart failure the dilation goes beyond the limits of aiding the strength of the contraction. It is very typical to see *pitting edema* in a woman with heart failure—her legs are swollen and a "pit" forms in the skin when you press your thumb down into it.

The sympathetic nervous system, which regulates tissues that aren't under our voluntary control, may respond to heart failure by increasing the rate of the heartbeat, a condition known as *tachycardia*. This sympathetic system overdrive may result in sweating, clammy skin, and possible arrhythmias. Fluid retention also occurs because of poor blood flow to the kidneys and other vital organs.

In some patients, the body's valiant attempt to compensate allows cardiac output to return to a normal level, either on its own, or after medication. For others, the heart "decompensates," which means that all its adaptive mechanisms still aren't enough to preserve cardiac output.

Heart failure can occur anywhere in the heart—left or right side or biventricular (when the pumping action of both ventricles is imparied).

Treatment. In cases where heart failure progresses rapidly, hospitalization may be required so that immediate measures can be taken to reduce salt and water in the body. Drug therapy with a derivative of digitalis called *digoxin* (Lanoxin) will stimulate the contractile ability of the heart. *Diuretics* such as Lasix will be prescribed to take fluid out of the body by permitting the kidneys to excrete more salt and water. Peripheral vasodilator drugs, or ACE inhibitors, such as enalapril (Vasotec) will widen blood vessels, making it easier for the heart to pump blood through them.

Because heart failure generally occurs in those whose hearts are already compromised by coronary artery disease, valvular disorders, or congenital problems, the best treatment is prevention. If you do have diagnosed heart disease, you should be under a physician's care. She can determine through regular examinations whether any procedures or surgery may be necessary to keep the heart pumping as it should.

Sudden Death

When death occurs within one hour of the onset of symptoms, this is known as "sudden death." Either blood flow to the heart is suddenly reduced, as in a heart attack, or an arrhythmia occurs, leading to ventricular fibrillation. A heart attack is not necessarily a prerequisite for sudden death however—the arrhythmia can be caused by ischemia from a clot, or atherosclerotic plaque. It can also occur in patients with heart failure.

Sudden death is not as common in women as in men. The Framingham Heart Study reported that it occurred in 37 percent of the women studied as compared to 46 percent of the men, and it occurred about twenty years later, in women aged sixty-five to seventy-four.

A Good Understanding of Your Disease Means Prompt Treatment

No matter what your condition, if you know what it is and how it can be diagnosed and treated, you are halfway toward a better health profile. It must also be said that although many varied disorders and malfunctions can occur, the heart is an incredibly potent organ, one that can often self-correct when necessary. And when it can't, we are fortunate to have the benefits of high-tech, innovative medical treatment that offers a stable future for those with heart disease. Given the proper attention, preventive care, and medication, you can and will improve the condition of your heart.

8

Diagnostic Testing

▽

We have come a long way from those days when the only diagnostic tools a doctor had at his command were a stethoscope and a blood pressure cuff. The innovative technology that exists today can pinpoint each of the various, complex issues in heart disease.

Women with heart disease of all types can benefit enormously from these state-of-the-art procedures and tests. When a doctor can see and measure the size, shape, and function of the heart, its various chambers and tissues, he becomes an informed advocate in your progress toward better heart health.

A woman with symptoms such as chest pain and shortness of breath *may* be suffering from coronary artery disease, but those symptoms could very well relate to some other problem. Until actual diagnostic studies have been completed, there is no way for a physician to tell what the source of the pain or difficulty in breathing might be. It's for this reason that your doctor may recommend any of the tests described in this chapter.

The costs of all these procedures vary, ranging from a few hundred dollars for a standard treadmill test in a doctor's office to several thousand dollars for a cardiac catheterization. However, if you have health insurance, some or all of the fees of both doctor and hospital will generally be paid.

Sister Catherine might not have survived without the specialized tests that revealed her coronary artery disease. She had lived with the pain in her chest for several years, not knowing whether it was serious or not, and not wanting to bother anyone about it.

"I told the Mother Superior it was the kind of thing that would come and go, and I thought, at seventy-seven, that it was natural. But eventually, we decided I should see the doctor about it. It was a good thing, too, because he sent me up for a cardiac catheterization at the hospital right around the corner from our church. Four days later, I had three bypasses. They'd found that one of my arteries was 100 percent blocked, one was 90 percent and one was 70 percent. They took a vein from my leg to make the graft, and of course that had to heal, too, along with my chest.

"I spent three months in cardiac rehabilitation. I made so many new friends when I was there—we'd have the same schedule and we'd be on the machines together. I used the treadmill, the arm ergometer, and the stationary bike while the nurses monitored my heart rate. They went through a whole nutritional program for me, since I'm a diabetic, and now it seems to me I never eat any fats, sugars or salt.

"I was fine until a month ago, when I started to feel the chest pain again. So I had a cardiac stress test (with a radionuclide tracer) to see how I was doing. My life has been saved at least twice by the tests I took."

How Does Your Physician Know What Tests to Administer?

The best care comes from the best doctor/patient relationship. If you have established this type of give and take with your physician (see Chapter 5), you are already on the road to learning what problems you may have and how they might be treated.

A woman who is having considerable symptoms of heart disease—angina, shortness of breath, blackouts—will obviously be concerned enough to seek medical attention. And once in a cardiologist's office, she will have access to all the diagnostic testing she needs.

But a woman who has no symptoms—and so many women have silent disease—may not seek help until it is too late. Because heart disease can hide so effectively, it is essential that every woman have a regular checkup once a year after the age of fifty so that any abnormalities in heart rate, cholesterol level, or blood pressure can be picked up. Some women have their first major checkup decades after the birth of their children just because they want to start an exercise program, or because they realize that they have a family history of heart disease and want to see what their risk factors are.

There isn't always a logical sequence to the order of testing, since not every procedure is relevant to every condition. Your doctor will deem appropriate whatever is indicated for your symptoms or lack of symptoms. The rule of thumb for any good diagnostician is that you work from noninvasive to invasive techniques. As each test proceeds, the doctor picks up more clues about what is going on in the body, which will determine the course of future treatment.

Decisions About Diagnostic Tests for Women

Women have not been treated as aggressively as men for heart disease, and so it is not surprising to learn that women often don't receive the number of sophisticated tests that men do, even when they display the same symptoms. Of course, since many types of female heart disease are asymptomatic, it would be prudent for every woman to have some basic tests that would be determined by her personal risk factors.

Whether you get the tests you need will usually depend on the recommendations of your doctor, the equipment available in your local hospital and whether they have the personnel to run them adequately, whether or not you have insurance that will pay for the tests, and certainly, your own attitude toward your care.

You know, if you are honest with yourself, that you may avoid having a mammogram because you're terrified of what the results might be. You may even avoid a monthly breast self-exam for fear of finding a lump. It's not uncommon to ignore or downplay symptoms when the issue at hand is having a test that may yield unpleasant results.

And so, women may receive less aggressive care because they tend to *request* less aggressive care. Typically, a woman will ask for medication to treat angina or high blood pressure or hypercholesterolemia and may stay on this regime sometimes long after its effectiveness is exhausted. Doctors are often willing to stick with the course of medication beyond the point where it could make a difference in a woman's condition. After all, everyone is sensitive these days about ordering expensive procedures, many of which are more difficult to evaluate for a woman than for a man.

So very often, although a man with angina might be promptly recommended for cardiac catheterization or balloon angioplasty, a woman might not get such care until it was overly apparent that medication was not alleviating her condition. As we've mentioned earlier, this might account for the higher death rates of women who do go through angioplasty and coronary bypass surgery.

So the fault for less aggressive treatment has to be equally shared. Doctor and patient must come to a clear understanding about why certain tests should or should not be ordered. Yes, it may be more comfortable to leave your doctor's office with a prescription and a pep talk, but in the long run, this may put you at greater risk.

You also have to look at your lifestyle and think about the way you expect to live in the future. If your major hobby is knitting, medications may maintain your heart in adequate shape. If you're a die-hard walker, it may be important to have angioplasty and try to open the blockages in your arteries. If you're a champion skier, possibly only bypass surgery will restore you to the life you wish to lead.

If you're taking a wait-and-see attitude, however, you may be jeopardizing your future, particularly if you happen to be on the threshold of a heart attack or you have a congenital condition that has grown more serious over the years. If you're not improving on medication alone, it is time to sit down with your physician and have a serious conversation about a new direction for care.

Which Basic Tests Are Right for You?

The diagnostic tests and therapeutic interventions that are available to you include:

NONINVASIVE DIAGNOSTIC TECHNIQUES
- physical examination
- blood pressure readings
- laboratory work (blood and urine tests)
- ECG
- exercise stress testing with or without radionuclide imaging or echocardiographic imaging
- chest X ray
- echocardiography
- Doppler echocardiography
- Holter monitor, loop recorders, and cardiobeepers
- MUGA
- MRI
- Tilt table study

THERAPEUTIC (INVASIVE) INTERVENTIONS
- cardiac catheterization and angiography
- EPS (electrophysiology study)
- balloon angioplasty (see Chapter 9)
- balloon valvuloplasty (see Chapter 9)
- open heart surgery

If you are a fifty-year-old woman with no symptoms, low risk factors, and no family history, you should still have a baseline ECG taken in your doctor's office along with your physical exam and blood-pressure check as well as routine laboratory blood and urine tests.

If you are fifty and have no symptoms, a few risk factors, and some family history of CHD, in addition to the above it would be wise to have an exercise stress test, possibly with echocardiographic imaging or a radionuclide tracer.

If you are fifty and are experiencing angina, you should certainly have all of the above tests. If your exercise stress test with echocardiography or the radionuclide tracer yielded positive results, your doctor might wish to order a cardiac catheterization.

The diagnostic process is very much like following a treasure map: the results of each test will tell your doctor where to go next. When there are missing clues, she can always order another, more specific test that will yield more definite answers.

Diagnostic Tests for Heart Disease

1. STETHOSCOPE AND BLOOD PRESSURE CUFF (SPHYGMOMANOMETER)

Purpose. The blood pressure cuff, by cutting off circulation in the arm and then releasing it, is able to determine the force of your blood as it washes against the arterial walls in each contraction and relaxation of the heart.

The stethoscope, a centuries-old device, magnifies the sound of your heartbeat. Each time you inhale and exhale, the earpieces of the stethoscope pick up the beat, any missed or irregular beats, and even the hiss of a heart murmur.

How It Is Performed. The blood pressure cuff contains a rubber bladder, which fills with air as the doctor pumps up the cuff. When the pressure in the bladder exceeds the pressure in the artery, the doctor will no longer be able to hear the heart beating. At this point, she will release the pressure until she hears the blood flowing in the vessel once again. This first sound, which registers the heart's contraction when blood is pumped into the arteries, is the *systolic* reading. This sound results from the turbulence generated as blood starts to enter the previously blocked artery.

As the doctor lets go of more air in the bladder, the sound of blood flow stops because the blood flow has become "smooth" or "laminar" again. At this point, the gauge will register the *diastolic* reading. A systolic to diastolic reading above 140/90 is classified as high blood pressure.

When heart disease is suspected, the physician may take pressure readings in both arms and legs. She will also listen to the heartbeat with a stethoscope not only around the heart and lungs, but also at the carotid artery in the neck.

The physical palpation (pressing) is also important. A physician will take pulses in both wrists, legs, and the carotid artery in the neck. Just feeling the chest area around the heart can indicate whether there's any enlargement.

2. LABORATORY WORK (BLOOD AND URINE ANALYSIS)

Purpose. A *urine sample* will detect a spillage of sugar, which might indicate diabetes, or red blood cells, which might indicate kidney damage.

Blood tests will be administered and analyzed for HDL and LDL cholesterol as well as triglycerides. Other blood samples will be analyzed for thyroid levels, since an overactive thyroid gland can cause palpitations.

3. ECG (ELECTROCARDIOGRAM)

Purpose. An ECG will show abnormalities in the electrical activity of the heart, certain arrhythmias, and sometimes, signs of ischemia (deficiency of blood supply to the heart).

How It Is Performed. As you lie on an examining table, twelve leads are attached to various areas on your chest, arms, and legs, secured by a type of gel that offers good conduction. Wires lead from the electrodes on your chest to the machine so that it can record your heart's electrical activity on graph paper.

What the Test Shows. The segments between each beat are represented by arcs and spikes on the paper. This pattern is charted by the letters P-QRS-T. The first arc, P, shows the atrial electrical activity. The second element, QRST, shows the ventricular electrical activity. Generally, the pattern looks like a flat segment up to the P wave, then a small wave, a spike from Q up to R and down to S, then a third flat segment (the ST segment), and a final T-wave.

An ischemic heart—where blood flow is restricted—will have a dip below baseline after the spike. Any abnormality in the waves, spikes, and segments can mean trouble. For example, if you do have coronary artery disease, dips or depressions in the ST segment may develop when you're exercising. By reproducing your symptoms on a treadmill test, the doctor will be able to pinpoint this dysfunctional area in a controlled situation.

The patterns made by the heartbeat on the graph paper can indicate disease and give warning of some possible cardiac event that might take place in the future. But it can also show the extent of damage from a heart attack that has already occurred. Sometimes a subsequent ECG is the only way to determine that a woman has had a "silent" heart attack.

Women's hearts often do not conform to the typical picture, however. It is harder to pinpoint coronary artery disease in women from just an ECG because the machine may not pick up arrhythmias or spasms that occur irregularly—and don't happen to occur when the machine is on.

Women often have slight abnormalities of their ST segments during stress testing—and this can cause a physician to read a healthy woman's ECG as abnormal. To avoid "false positives," many women are now being tested on a treadmill with some type of imaging—either echocardiographic or thallium.

4. CHEST X RAY

Purpose. The view of the heart on an X-ray screen shows some structural abnormalities and whether or not it is enlarged. Congenital conditions may also be picked up on an X ray.

How It Is Performed. A technician will have you stand against the X-ray monitor at different angles, and you will be asked to hold your breath briefly as each picture is taken. This procedure delivers a very small amount of radiation, which is not at all hazardous to your health unless you are pregnant. If you know that you might be pregnant, you should not receive X-ray radiation, as it can damage the unborn fetus.

5. EXERCISE STRESS TESTING
   Purpose. To examine the heart's function under physical stress. A stress test would be given to evaluate chest pain or arrhythmias, or to assess cardiac function, particularly after heart attack or heart surgery.
   How It Is Performed. A typical stress test is given on a treadmill in the doctor's office. Leads are attached to various areas on your chest that hook up to the electrodes on the ECG machine. A baseline ECG, heart rate, and blood pressure are obtained. You begin walking, and gradually your heart is put under increasing stress from a steeper inclination and faster speed of the treadmill. After you reach your target heart rate, the machine is slowed, and the heart's capacity for recovery is then measured.

In individuals with cardiovascular disease, this test may trigger arrhythmias or angina.

Stress Testing in Women. A stress test simply may not be as reliable in women as in men. If a physician sees abnormalities on a middle-aged man's ECG as he walks uphill on a treadmill, and this man has been suffering from angina, he can pretty safely say that his patient has some form of heart disease. It is true that in 10 percent of all cases—male and female—the standard treadmill test gives false positive results. But the sensitivity and predictive valve of future cardiac trouble is much better in men than women—the test gives men a diagnostic sensitivity and specificity of 80 and 74 percent respectively, whereas the percentages for women are 76 and 64 percent.

The other problem in gauging the value of this test is that women with heart disease don't always have the same symptoms as men. With typical angina, the predictive value of a positive exercise test is about 83 percent, however this value drops to 50 percent if a woman has atypical angina or no symptoms at all.

For this reason, several variations on the exercise test are often recommended for women.

6. EXERCISE STRESS TESTING WITH RADIOACTIVE TRACER OR ECHOCARDIOGRAPHIC IMAGING

Purpose. To examine the heart's function under physical stress, using either a radioactive tracer or echocardiographic imaging. These two variations on the treadmill stress test give finer sensitivity and a more accurate predictive value of future cardiovascular problems in women.

Stress testing with exercise **thallium myocardial perfusion scintigraphy** correctly excludes false positives in 85 percent of cases, greatly improving diagnostic accuracy in women over a plain stress test. The only problem with thallium is that it does not always allow good views of the heart if it is obscured by breast implants or lung disorders. But a newer isotope, **Cardiolite (technetium Tc-99m sestamibi),** seems to resolve this problem. The combination of X ray, ECG, and exercise thallium or Cardiolite scintigraphy gives a doctor a clear picture of each patient.

How the Thallium or Cardiolite Tests Are Performed. These medications are first injected into your bloodstream while you are resting, and a special camera X-rays your heart. (The amount of radiation you receive is about equal to that in a CT scan.) Then, at a second visit to the lab, more dye is injected as you are walking on a treadmill, with leads attached to electrodes that connect to an ECG. The two different results are then compared so that your physician can measure the amount of blood flowing through the heart at rest and under stress. If any part of the heart isn't receiving thallium, that means it is also not receiving enough blood. This test is approximately 90 percent accurate in diagnosing coronary artery disease in both men and women.

Many physicians feel that a stress test with **echocardiogram imaging** is the best choice for a woman with angina. It is more accurate than plain stress testing and involves no exposure to radiation, as do the thallium and Cardiolite tests. It can also "see" through breast implants, which may obscure the results of the radionuclide tests. (See below for the description of echocardiogram imaging.)

7. IV PERSANTINE-THALLIUM TEST

Purpose. To examine the heart's function under physical stress when the patient is not able to exercise.

How It Is Performed. You lie on an examining table and the ECG leads will be placed on various areas of your chest around and over the heart. The leads will then be attached to the ECG machine. A camera with an X-ray screen is positioned near you to take pictures of your heart.

The cardiologist will then insert an intravenous line in your arm so that two medications can be administered. The first drug, Persantine, will take about four minutes to enter your bloodstream. This medication will dilate your coronary arteries, just as though you were exercising. After this, you will receive the thallium, the radioactive dye that can be detected by the X-ray camera used to take pictures of your heart.

8. ECHOCARDIOGRAM

Purpose. This test indicates how your heart and valves are working and the size of your various chambers. It can also detect muscular abnormalities from hypertension or cardiomyopathy (disease of the heart muscles).

How It Is Performed. You may be familiar with this test if you had a sonogram when you were pregnant. An echocardiogram uses sound waves to create two- or three-dimensional images of the heart. The waves bounce or "echo" off the surface of the heart, creating patterns of the chambers and valves that are then translated into electronic images.

While you lie on your side on an examining table, a technician moves a wand or transducer over your chest. The transducer picks up the sound waves from your cardiac structures, which can be visualized on a video screen and recorded on videotape.

Types of Echocardiography. The conventional echocardiogram uses a two-dimensional ultrasound beam to look at cardiac chamber size and function. Most types of valve problems can be examined with this technique—it is possible to see how the leaflets close and open. It can show whether valves are thickened, and whether they have the correct number of leaflets. The test is also useful for diagnosing pericardial disease, pulmonary hypertension, aneurysms, congestive heart failure, and damage from a heart attack.

Another type of echo (sometimes performed in conjunction with two-dimensional readings) includes use of the Doppler measurement, which evaluates the *blood flow, velocity,* and *direction* of the blood through the valves and chambers. This study gives a physician a good idea of how severely a valve is malfunctioning—that is, how badly narrowed it is and how much leaking you have.

An echocardiogram can be performed on a patient during their exercise stress test, however the accuracy of the reading depends on the experience of the interpreter. Again, the reading on an elderly, frail woman who may have trouble performing the exercise could read differently from that of a young, active woman. It may also be more difficult to read a test performed on a woman with lung disease or breast implants, which can obscure the clarity of the ultrasound pictures. Large breasts are not usually a problem—the ultrasound can "see" through fat quite well.

9. HOLTER MONITOR

Purpose. To record any unusual cardiac event that might take place over a twenty-four-hour period using a continuous microchip recording of the heart's electrical activity.

How It Is Performed. You wear a portapak (about the size of a Walkman radio) around your neck or waist or over your shoulder, and wires are attached to your chest. Your heart and physical activity are recorded over the course of a day, and the two are compared to analyze rhythm and changes in the ECG. Since some activity can bring on arrhythmias or coronary artery spasm, you'll be asked to keep a diary of your day's activities, which can be matched up to the results of the Holter recording.

10. LOOP MONITOR, CARDIOBEEPER

Purpose. To diagnose an unusual cardiac event that might occur rarely, in a time period greater than twenty-four hours.
How It Is Performed. Worn like a Holter monitor, the loop monitor erases the electrical activity that has just passed every five minutes when it "loops" around to the beginning of the tape again. When an irregular rhythm or some other abnormal occurrence like an imminent blackout is in progress, you must depress the button that records the event and depress it a second time when the event is over. The advantage of the loop monitor is that if you experience some abnormality only every three months, it can successfully be caught on tape.

The cardiobeeper can be carried like a regular phone beeper on your belt or in your purse. If you feel dizzy or are having palpitations, you place it on your chest and a recording is made of the event. You can send this recording over the telephone to your physician.

11. CARDIAC CATHETERIZATION

Purpose. To determine whether there are blockages in the coronary arteries and/or to find the source of your chest pain. A catheterization might be ordered if you are having unstable angina or angina at a very low level of exercise or an abnormal stress test, a recent heart attack, or heart failure.

There are some risks involved. Because this procedure involves passing a catheter through a blood vessel and possibly dislodging plaque, there is a one in three thousand chance of a stroke, heart attack, or sudden death. Some individuals may have an allergic reaction to the dye used in the procedure. And individuals with kidney disease may be adversely affected by the passage of the dye out of the body, since it must travel through the kidneys to be excreted in the urine.

Preparation for the Test. You will usually have an ECG and blood work the day of the catheterization. After this, you will be brought into the catheterization lab and lightly sedated. You'll be lying on an X-ray table with a large camera over your head. Your heart will be monitored on an ECG, and several leads will be attached from your chest to the ECG machine. Blood pressure and heart rate will be continuously recorded during the procedure. The physician will inject a local anesthetic at the site in your brachial (arm) or femoral (groin) artery where the catheter will be inserted. This may sting a little.

How It Is Performed. A catheterization and angiogram (or arteriogram) is performed by passing a thin plastic tube into a blood vessel in the arm or groin which leads into the heart. A contrast dye is infused into the catheter that outlines blood flow on X-ray motion pictures, known as angiograms or arteriograms. By looking at the progress of the blood through the arteries, it is possible to tell whether there are blockages or narrowings and how serious they are. It is also possible to measure heart valve function with this procedure.

Women and Catheterization. Women's chest pain is often more elusive than men's and isn't always caused by blockages of plaque. The Framingham Heart Study reported that 50 percent of women with chest pain had little or no evidence of obstruction on arteriogram, as compared with 17 percent of men. Many physicians feel that this test is overused, certainly in men, and that noninvasive discovery of coronary artery disease is more cost effective. But if you are having pain that is not being alleviated by medication, if you have already had an abnormal noninvasive test, this procedure should be done. Nothing will show the exact locations of blockages like a catheterization.

12. EPS (ELECTROPHYSIOLOGY STUDY)

Purpose. To determine the cause of arrhythmias.

How It Is Performed. This invasive test is similar to a catheterization, and you will be lightly sedated before it. An insulated tube that contains temporary pacemaker wires is passed through your arm, groin, or neck into your heart. By viewing the electrical impulses generated by your heart on a fluoroscope (similar to an X ray) screen, and by changing your heart's natural "pacing" with the wires, your physician will be able to measure how electrical impulses flow through your heart during a heartbeat.

In order to test your heart's capacity, the electrophysiologist will purposely change the impulses directed toward your heart so that you may skip beats or feel your heart race. By mimicking the arrhythmias you experience, your physician will be able to determine ways to treat your problem.

13. MRI (MAGNETIC RESONANCE IMAGING)

Purpose. To make detailed images of the heart using a powerful magnet and radio waves that bounce images off the internal organs. This test is useful to diagnose tumors, pericardial disease, and congenital defects.

How It Is Performed. You lie on a table, encased in a long tube that is lined with a powerful, superconductive magnet. As you lie inside the hollow cylinder of the machine for the next hour, you must be completely still. You can listen to music on headphones if you wish.

This noninvasive diagnosis targets specific cells of your body and magnetically changes their energy output. This may create a clanging noise that is only alarming if you aren't prepared for it. The powerful magnet can measure the distribution of atoms in the heart and produce an image of the tissue on a computer screen in the adjoining room.

The typical CT scan is too slow to give an accurate picture of the heart arteries because the heart moves with each heartbeat. However, a **gated MRI** or **rapid CT-scan** can look at the arteries. *Gated* means that the machine breaks the action of the heart into ten specific cardiac cycles, which can reveal the specific source and severity of your dysfunction.

14. MUGA (MULTIPLE-GATED ACQUISITION TEST)

Purpose. To see if your heart has been damaged by a previous heart attack or infection, as well as to evaluate heart muscle function in patients with heart failure.

How It Is Performed. A radioisotope that can "tag" certain blood cells is injected into the brachial artery in your arm. This special tag then proceeds into the chambers of your heart, where it can highlight the various areas, and they can be photographed by a special X-ray camera.

15. TILT-TABLE STUDY

Purpose. To determine causes of dizziness or blackouts.

How It Is Performed. You lie flat on a table in a darkened room, and the position of the table is tilted to mimic what happens when your body goes from prone to upright. Your blood pressure and heart rate are monitored throughout. Although the body's job is to regulate its alterations in posture automatically, this test will show whether your system is not adjusting properly. The malfunction might be caused by mitral valve prolapse or by a vasovagal irregularity—the response of the nervous system to the body's realignment.

Looking Inside the Heart

The high-tech procedures outlined in this chapter can offer astounding insights into every form of heart disease. But a test can only piece out the puzzle for a physician and point the way to possible treatment. The more you know about your diagnosis, the more comfortable you can feel about decisions you and your physician make with regard to treatment.

In the next chapter, we will learn exactly what can—and can't—be done to treat heart disease with medications, procedures, and surgery.

9

Managing Heart Disease with
Medication and Surgery

∇

If you have already been diagnosed with heart disease, you can't ignore your condition anymore. And regardless of what you think, feel, or fear about your future, there are many options open to you. You and your physician must consider all appropriate courses of action and then decide on a workable treatment plan.

Rose was, for years, one of the walking wounded. She was very sick but refused to admit it.

"Nobody ever told me that if you've got a pain that feels like indigestion, it could be your heart and you could need an operation," Rose said. "I remember this one Christmas Day, I was hurting so bad I almost couldn't deliver my presents. If I'd known I was close as a whisper to a heart attack, I would have gone home and went to bed. But I kept going from one relative to the next till I nearly fell down. My family wanted me in the hospital, but I was so stubborn I just said no, I'll manage.

"The next morning, I went to church, still wheezing so bad they could hear me up at the altar. But it was a good thing I went, because one of the women there knew Dr. Ross. I got to her just in time and never did have that heart attack. She knew that a bypass operation was the only thing that would save me."

At sixty-four, Rose is now an active, healthy survivor of bypass surgery. She blatantly refused to believe she was ill when all signs pointed to it.

Her father died of a heart attack at a young age, and she has diabetes and is hypertensive. Since her surgery she's been able to stay within normal range with medication and a low-fat diet of good fresh foods. She found a treadmill at Good Will for fifteen dollars and uses it about three times a week.

Her church is her greatest support. Even when she's worrying a lot about her family, she can find solace in prayer, and this really reduces her stress.

And since that fateful Christmas Day, she has another asset. She now knows the value of paying attention to herself. "If I was to tell anyone else what good came out of this," she says, "it's to think twice before you say you just have indigestion. Go to the doctor! Don't put it off! It could save your life."

Why didn't Rose realize that she was extremely ill and needed help? As a licensed practical nurse who had worked at hospitals as a young woman, she should have suspected that she suffered from more than indigestion. Thank goodness her family and friends insisted that she receive real medical attention and got her into surgery in time.

Should Your Condition Be Medically Managed?

Treating heart disease is a complex matter, and what works for one patient doesn't necessarily work for another. Once you've been diagnosed and know exactly what type of problem you have, the options about what to do start to narrow.

A man with heart disease often has a massive heart attack as his first symptom—and therefore he gets rushed into surgery. Drastic emergency measures have to be taken to save his life. A woman, however, typically can be medically managed for years. She may suffer tolerable bouts of angina for decades, but as long as she responds well to her various drugs (for high blood pressure, cholesterol, coagulation, arrhythmias, etc.), her physician won't refer her to a surgeon. Anyway, many women protest hotly if an operation is advised. Women just don't want to take time out to go to the hospital—they're needed too badly at home. And for some women, surgery can be dangerous or inadvisable. What are some reasons that a woman would not be a good candidate for surgery and therefore should be kept on medication?

- Her coronary artery disease has not advanced enough, and medical management is keeping it under control.
- She is a surgical risk because her CAD is too advanced, with disease throughout the coronary arteries.
- She has already had extensive damage to her heart muscle.
- She has other medical complications and illnesses.
- She has refused surgical treatment and is willing to change her lifestyle radically with a very restricted low-fat diet, a program of daily exercise, and stress reduction.

Medication in and of itself doesn't cure heart disease—what it can do is alter body chemistry and ease the function of the heart. The irony, however, is that if a woman grows older on heart medication and her condition worsens over the years, it may be too late once she's taken to surgery to repair the long-term damage.

How long should *you* stay on medication? As long as you and your physician agree that the drugs are helping your condition, there's no reason to stop.

Because you will be taking several drugs at a time, vigilance about when and how you take the drugs is essential. You and your physician should review the particular drugs and dosages you're taking at least once a year, and sooner if you're having side effects or the drugs aren't doing the job they're supposed to.

Which Medications Will Keep a Woman's Heart Healthy?

There are several varieties of drugs that are common for patients with heart disease. Typically, doctors prescribe:

1. Oral or Transdermal Nitroglycerin. For years, the first line of treatment for angina has been a nitroglycerin tablet under the tongue. The twenty-four-hour transdermal nitroglycerin patch, worn like an estrogen patch (see Chapter 6), is useful for those with chronic angina.

The function of this drug is to dilate the arteries and veins so that there is improved blood supply to the heart, which consequently won't have to work so hard. Of course, since the blood vessels throughout the entire body are dilated, this drug can cause headaches. It may also have the effect of lowering blood pressure rapidly, which can make you feel as though you're going to faint.

Although nitroglycerin has its drawbacks, it is certainly a first-line medication for angina—although it won't stop a heart attack that's already begun.

2. Diuretics. All three types of diuretics (thiazide, loop, and potassium-sparing) act by reducing salt and water in the body. They are used in conjunction with other antihypertensive medications that tend to make you retain fluid. They are also used to treat congestive heart failure.

3. Beta-Blockers. These drugs lower the heart's demand for oxygen under stress. A person with high blood pressure, for example, may develop angina when particularly upset—a beta-blocker blocks the effect of the sympathetic nervous system on the heart muscle and takes the stress off the arteries.

4. Calcium Channel Blockers. These drugs prevent spasm in the coronary arteries by lowering the amount of calcium flowing into the muscle cells located in the walls of the coronary arteries. They may be used alone or in combination with beta-blockers.

In addition, depending on your needs, your physician may prescribe drugs to lower your *cholesterol* and *triglycerides,* drugs to control *arrhythmias, vasodilators* (drugs to dilate blood vessels), *anticoagulants, antiplatelet medication,* and *hormone replacement therapy.*

If you are currently experiencing side effects from your medications that you find uncomfortable or troublesome, don't be shy. Talk to your doctor about the dosage and the medication itself—there may be a good alternative that won't cause you such distress. Never stop taking your medication abruptly—by doing so you might put your body into a chemically imbalanced state. In addition, rapid withdrawal from a powerful drug can cause additional side effects.

Below are some of the most common medications prescribed for heart disease.

Cholesterol- and Triglyceride-Lowering Drugs

All of these types of drugs must be used in conjunction with a low-fat, low-cholesterol diet and a regular exercise program.

Drugs: Questran (cholestyramine) or Colestid (colestipol).

Purpose: Binds bile acids in the intestine and prevents their reabsorption into bloodstream. This increases excretion of cholesterol.

Side Effects: Constipation, indigestion, gallstones.

Interactions: May decrease effectiveness of beta-blockers, thiazide diuretics, anticoagulants, seizure medication, certain antibiotics, and Digoxin.

Drugs: Atromid-S (clofibrate) or Lopid (gemfibrozil).

Purpose: To prevent production of triglycerides and cholesterol in the liver. Lopid raises HDLs and reduces triglycerides.

Side Effects: Diarrhea, nausea, vomiting.

Interactions: Increases effectiveness of anticoagulants.

Drugs: Mevacor (Lovastatin), Pravachol, Zocor.

Purpose: These drugs, which are classified as HMG co-A reductase inhibitors, reduce LDL, total cholesterol, and triglycerides and raise HDL by blocking the formation of cholesterol in the liver.

Side Effects: Headache, muscle soreness, liver function abnormalities.

Interactions: Increases effectiveness of anticoagulants. Should not be used with gemfibrozil or large doses of niacin.

Drug: Nicolar (niacin)
Purpose: Reduces production of LDLs.
Side Effects: Flushing, tingling, headache.

Interactions: Increases effectiveness of some hypertensive drugs; decreases effectiveness of some diabetic drugs.

Antihypertensive Drugs

DIURETICS
THIAZIDE DIURETICS (These drugs are long acting—they are also less powerful than loop diuretics.)

Drugs: Hydrodiuril, Hydrochlorthiazide, Maxide, Esidrix.
Purpose: To lower blood pressure. Causes the kidney to increase urine excretion, so the body can eliminate more salt and water. The loss of salt will lower blood pressure in hypertensive patients.
Side Effects: Potassium loss, which makes for a dry mouth, increased thirst, mood changes, muscle cramps, nausea, fatigue.
Interactions: Increases effects of other hypertensive medications; raises lithium levels.

LOOP DIURETICS (These drugs work quickly, causing you to excrete a lot of urine within a few hours of taking the medication. Often used for people with kidney as well as heart disease.)

Drugs: Lasix, Bumex.
Purpose: To lower blood pressure. Causes kidney to increase urine excretion and the body to eliminate salt and water. The loss of salt will lower blood pressure in hypertensive patients.

Side Effects: Dizziness, potassium loss, which causes dry mouth, mood changes, muscle cramps, nausea, fatigue.
Interactions: Increases effects of other hypertensive drugs.

POTASSIUM-SPARING DIURETICS (These are the weakest of the three varieties of diuretics but are usually effective after two or three days of use.)

Drugs: Aldactone, Midamor, Dyrenium.
Purpose: To lower blood pressure (same as other diuretics).
Side Effects: Nausea, dry mouth, muscle cramps, diarrhea, vomiting, sweating.
Interactions: Increases effect of other antihypertensive drugs.

BETA-BLOCKERS
B1 SELECTIVE BETA-ADRENERGIC BLOCKERS (works on receptor sites in the heart only).

Drugs: Lopressor, Tenormin.
Purpose: To lower blood pressure and relieve angina by blocking action of sympathetic nervous system, slowing the heart rate.
Side Effects: Dizziness, fatigue, may cause wheezing or congestive heart failure.
Interactions: Increases effects of antihypertensive drugs, sedatives, tranquilizers, and others.

NONSELECTIVE BETA-ADRENERGIC BLOCKERS (works on receptor sites in the heart, lungs, and blood vessels).

Drugs: Inderal, Blocadren, Levatol, Corgard.
Purpose: To lower blood pressure and give preventive care against heart attacks by slowing heart rate, blocking the effects of adrenaline.
Side Effects: May cause wheezing and shortness of breath, since it works on receptor sites in the lungs. Also, dizziness, sleep disturbance, fatigue, decreased sexual desire in women (Inderal has been known to cause erectile dysfunction in men).

Interactions: Increases effects of other antihypertensive drugs, sedatives, tranquilizers, and others. May not be appropriate for diabetics, as it blocks the symptoms of hypoglycemia (low blood sugar).

ALPHA and BETA-ADRENERGIC BLOCKERS (A newer variety of beta-blocker that has fewer side effects than beta-blockers.)

Drugs: Normodyne, Trandate.
Purpose: To reduce blood pressure.
Side Effects: Dizziness, sleep disturbances, sexual dysfunction.
Interactions: Increases the effect of diuretics.

CALCIUM CHANNEL BLOCKERS (Calcium Antagonists)
Drugs: Cardizem, Calan, Procardia.
Purpose: To lower blood pressure, relieve angina, and treat atrial flutter by preventing calcium from flowing into the cells of the heart and blood vessels. They also relax the blood vessels and reduce the force of the heart's contractions.
Side Effects: Headache, ankle edema. Cardizem may slow heart rate, but Procardia will increase it.
Interactions: Increases effect of other antihypertensive drugs, may cause excess slowing of heart rate in patients on Digoxin or beta-blockers.

Vasodilators

These drugs widen blood vessels, which lowers the resistance to blood flow through the cardiovascular system.

ACE (ANGIOTENSIN-CONVERTING ENZYME) INHIBITORS
Drugs: Capoten, Vasotec.
Purpose: To lower blood pressure and treat heart failure by inhibiting the release of the enzyme angiotensin, which constricts blood vessels.
Side Effects: Loss of taste, coughing, dizziness, constipation.

Interactions: Increases effects of other antihypertensive drugs; should not be used with potassium supplements or potassium-sparing diuretics.

PERIPHERAL VASODILATORS
Drugs: Apresoline, Hydralazine.
Purpose: To treat hypertension and heart failure by dilating blood vessels and decreasing resistance to blood flow.
Side Effects: Diarrhea, headache, nausea, heart palpitations.
Interactions: Increases effect of other antihypertensives and diuretics.

ALPHA-1-ADRENERGIC BLOCKERS
Drugs: Minipress, Hytrin.
Purpose: To treat hypertension and heart failure by suppressing blood vessel receptors usually stimulated by adrenaline to contract the vessels.
Side Effects: Dizziness, edema, headache.
Interactions: Increases effect of other antihypertensives, especially beta-blockers.

NITRATES
Drugs: Ismo; in emergencies, nitroglycerine administered under the tongue.
Purpose: To relieve angina by widening veins and arteries, thus lowering blood pressure.
Side Effects: Low blood pressure, headache.
Interactions: Increases effects of other antihypertensive drugs.

CENTRAL ALPHA-ADRENERGIC AGONISTS
Drugs: Aldomet, Catapres, Wytensin, Tenex.
Purpose: To stimulate brain receptors that cause blood pressure to lower.
Side Effects: Headache, drowsiness.
Interactions: Increases effects of antihypertensive and anticoagulant drugs.

PERIPHERAL ADRENERGIC BLOCKERS
Drugs: Reserpine, Hylorel, Ismelin.
Purpose: To lower blood pressure by inhibiting the release of a stress hormone, thus reducing tension in blood vessel walls.
Side Effects: Dry mouth, dizziness, diarrhea, loss of appetite, sexual dysfunction, slow heartbeat, angina, depression.
Interactions: Increases effects of other antihypertensives and sedatives.

Antiarrhythmia Drugs

These medications either slow down or eradicate abnormal heartbeats. All medications in this category are very powerful and must be carefully titrated for the individual patient. Some of these drugs speed up electrical conduction in the heart; others affect particular areas of the conduction system in specific ways.

Drugs: Lanoxin.
Purpose: To strengthen heart muscle contractions and stabilize rate and rhythm of the heartbeat.
Side Effects: (Usually result from toxicity) excess slowing of heart rate, nausea, visual disturbances.
Interactions: With beta-blockers and calcium blockers. Both can cause excess slowing of heart rate.

Drugs: Norpace, Procan, Quinidine, Tambocor.
Purpose: To treat irregular heartbeat by various effects on the electrical system of the heart.
Side Effects: Diarrhea, loss of appetite, dry mouth, nausea, vomiting.
Interactions: Increases effectiveness of antihypertensives, anti-coagulants, and other arrhythmics; Quinidine raises Digoxin levels.

Blood-Clotting Drugs

These drugs prevent the formation of blood clots. The danger of a blood clot is twofold: first, it stops the free flow of blood through a vessel and second, it can become dislodged and travel through the bloodstream (an *embolism*).

ANTICOAGULANTS

Drugs: Heparin (administered intravenously); Coumadin (warfarin) administered orally.

Purpose: Heparin prevents clots from forming by reducing production of **fibrin,** a protein that assists in the clotting process. Coumadin blocks the formation of clotting factors that depend on vitamin K.

Side Effects: Bruising, bleeding.

Interactions: Interactions with many different types of drugs, prescription, and over-the-counter. Your physician must be informed about all other drugs you are taking. Do not consume alcohol if you are taking these drugs. The dosage of Heparin must be carefully titrated—higher-than-average doses have been shown to increase risk of stroke.

THROMBOLYTIC DRUGS

Drugs: Streptase (streptokinase), tPA, Activase.

Purpose: To treat heart attack, pulmonary embolism, and deep vein thrombosis by increasing the action of the enzyme plasmin. This effectively dissolves a clot by breaking up the strands of fibrin that hold the blood platelets together.

Side Effects: Excessive bleeding—this can be extremely dan- · gerous.

Interactions: Can interact with any other drug that affects blood platelet activity.

ANTIPLATELET MEDICATION

In the Aspirin Myocardial Infarction Study, no clear benefit in taking a daily aspirin was shown on survival rates for women as it was for men, but the females tested were older and at higher risk. There is usually no harm—and may be a great deal of good—in taking a daily aspirin in order to cause the platelets to be less sticky and give them less opportunity to adhere to the blood vessel membranes.

Drugs: Aspirin, Ticlid.

Purpose: Prevention of heart attack and stroke by decreasing the tendency of the clotting cells (platelets) to stick together.

Side Effects: Heartburn, ulcers, ringing in the ears.

Interactions: Increases effects of anticoagulants.

Hormone Replacement Therapy

Drug: Premarin (estrogen).

Purpose: To prevent heart disease in postmenopausal women by elevating HDL cholesterol, widening blood vessels, and making them more elastic.

Side Effects: Weight gain, bloating, elevated blood pressure. Contraindicated in any woman with estrogen-dependent cancer. Certain studies indicate that long-term use may increase your risk of breast or endometrial cancer, gallstones, kidney, or liver disease.

Interactions: None.

Drug: Provera (progestin) if needed for women who still have a uterus.

Purpose: To balance hormonal environment of endometrium in a postmenopausal woman who is taking estrogen.

Side Effects: Bloating, sore breasts, mood changes, depression, nausea.

Interactions: None.

(See Chapter 6 for a full discussion of hormone replacement therapy.)

Are You a Good Candidate for Angioplasty?

There may come a point when it will be clear that some treatment other than drugs is necessary. If medical management has not relieved your pain and other symptoms, if your angina is getting worse, if you experience difficulty breathing, you and your physician will need to discuss *balloon angioplasty*, also known as PTCA—percutaneous transluminal coronary angioplasty. (*Percutaneous* means "through the skin," and *transluminal* means "inside the artery.")

Balloon Angioplasty

This procedure was developed in Switzerland by a Dr. Andreas Gruentzig in 1977 as an alternative to bypass surgery. Although it is invasive, it does not involve cutting and stitching the heart. A patient too weak and frail to survive open heart surgery may be able to get the same relief from PTCA. The procedure starts out as a cardiac catheterization (see Chapter 8), and uses a small catheter that has a small balloon on the end of it.

WHAT ARE THE CONTRAINDICATIONS FOR PTCA?

Your medical history, a treadmill test, and your coronary angiogram (see Chapter 8) will determine how good a candidate you are for this procedure. Ideally, the narrowing in your artery should be less than 10 millimeters in length and not involve the point where two major vessels meet. If your lesion or narrowing is in a particularly difficult location, you will not be recommended for this procedure. Other reasons that you might not be recommended for PTCA include:

- an excessive number of stenoses (narrowings) in one or several vessels
- disease in the left main coronary artery.

In these cases, your physician will undoubtedly not wish to try "halfway" measures but will instead recommend coronary by-pass surgery (see below).

Preparation Before the Procedure. Prior to the procedure, you will have an ECG and routine blood tests. You may be shaved around the site of your femoral artery (in the groin) or brachial artery (in the arm) where the catheter will be inserted. An intravenous needle will be placed in a vein in your hand or arm so that medications and fluids can be given to you quickly. Just before you go up to the catheterization laboratory, you'll be given a mild sedative to help you relax.

The Catheterization Laboratory. The PTCA will take one or two hours, and the procedure is quite similar to cardiac catheterization (see page 157, Chapter 8). You'll be lying on an X-ray table, with a large camera over your head. The staff will wear lead suits, since they do these procedures all the time and can't risk the amount of radiation they'd receive daily. However you shouldn't worry about your own exposure—it is minimal for one procedure.

Your heart will be monitored on an ECG, and several leads will be attached from your chest to the machine. The physician will inject a local anesthetic at the site in your femoral artery where the catheter will be inserted. This may sting a little.

How Is the Procedure Done? The physician will thread the catheter up your femoral or brachial artery. A small introducer sheath will be inserted, and then the long flexible catheter will go in through the sheath.

Your physician will position the catheter at the opening of the coronary artery, and a contrast dye will be injected that follows the blood flow through the heart. You and your doctor can watch the progress of the dye on the video screen. The place where the dye stops is the location of the obstruction. Then the physician will advance the guide wire inside the catheter until the balloon is inside the narrowed segment. As the balloon tip reaches the site, the doctor manually inflates it, filling it with the contrast dye and stretching the walls of the artery. You may feel a sensation of angina as the balloon temporarily blocks the artery.

As the balloon is inflated, the plaque is compressed and sometimes split, opening the narrowed artery. Your physician may deflate and inflate the balloon several times in order to compress the plaque most effectively. If the balloon she has selected is too small to do the job, she may exchange it over a guide wire for a larger balloon.

At the end of the angioplasty, the physician will remove the balloon and take more X-ray pictures of the artery so that she can see that blood flow has improved.

Anya, who was sixty-nine when she had her angioplasty, said she was very apprehensive about it when it was described to her. ".I just couldn't imagine what it would feel like. And I think I was so nervous, I started having chest pains right there. But the doctor said it was because every time she blew up the balloon, the artery was blocked for a few seconds. She had her technician give me some pain medication and told me to breathe. Then she said, 'Mrs. Hanssen, this is when I give you the lecture about smoking cigarettes.' I was so surprised, I started laughing, right there on the table. But it made an impression, all right! I haven't had a cigarette since that day, though I've wanted to."

After the Procedure. You'll be taken back to your room and asked to lie still for a few hours while your blood pressure and heartbeat are constantly monitored. You'll be given Heparin (an anticoagulant) intravenously and asked to drink a lot of fluids so that your kidneys will be able to pass the contrast dye out of your body. The sheath will be left in place for six hours or possibly overnight. You'll probably have some pain in your leg or arm, and you may have some mild chest pain for a few hours after PTCA. You'll be able to get out of bed and walk within twelve to twenty-four hours. You can go home one or two days after the procedure.

As the blood vessel heals over the next few weeks, the dispersed plaque forms something akin to scar tissue. Smooth muscle cells grow in over the plaque to line the vessel walls.

What Are the Risks of This Procedure? As with regular catheterization, there is always some danger to inserting a catheter into an arm or leg. With angioplasty, there is a 1 to 3 percent chance that the vessel will close up during or immediately after the procedure, necessitating an immediate bypass operation. Often, even when the physician feels that angioplasty is appropriate, the blockage may be too massive for the catheter to dilate, in which case a bypass may then be recommended. It is very important, therefore, that you have this procedure done in a hospital where open heart surgery is routinely performed. You certainly can't afford the time to be transferred to a different facility should an emergency bypass be necessary.

How Successful Is PTCA in Women? In a report from the PTCA Registry of the National Heart, Lung and Blood Institute, published in *Circulation* and *The American Journal of Cardiology,* 1984 and 1985, it was found that women undergoing this procedure were typically older and had more unstable angina than men. The procedure was considered risky for a small individual with smaller arteries, which might tear as the balloon (developed with a man's larger vessels in mind) was inflated. Only six months after the procedure, 30 percent of the angioplasties had failed (this statistic is equally true for men). The complication rates were higher than for men.

But now, ten years later, the overall complication rate has decreased, although the failure rate after six months stands at 30 percent. In the past few years, smaller balloons have been developed to use in a woman's smaller blood vessels. In long-term follow-ups, women actually did better than men. If their angioplasties held up beyond the six-month marker, they had less restenosis and a higher survival rate. This might have something to do with their renewed motivation to stick to healthier eating and exercising.

But many fewer women than men are recommended for the procedure, even today. In 1992, there were 259,000 angioplasties performed in this country, and only 82,000 of them were done on women. But it is still less traumatic to the body than open heart surgery and is therefore the better first option for a woman with one- or two-vessel disease.

The degree of experience of your cardiologist is also a factor. Be sure you ask how many angioplasties she has performed in the past and what her success rate is with the procedure. The American College of Cardiology and the American Heart Association suggest that you should only seek this type of treatment from a physician who has performed at least 125 angioplasties and been the primary physician on the procedure team in about half of those.

Angioplasty with a Stent. If the vessel does collapse after angioplasty, all may not be lost. An **acute closure** of the vessel can be treated with a device called a **stent,** which will keep the artery open so that blood can continue to flow through it.

A stent is something like a bridge made of surgical-grade stainless steel that is loaded on the balloon catheter. It travels with the balloon to the obstruction in the vessel. The physician then inflates the balloon, and as it expands, so does the stent. The balloon is then deflated and removed, leaving the stent compressed into the blood vessel wall. Over the next days and weeks, scar tissue grows over it, keeping it in place.

Is the stent better than regular angioplasty? Not necessarily. The real gauge is the size of the vessel being worked on—the larger the vessel, the better the chance that the stent will hold up. But remember that women's vessels are generally smaller. Blockages in bypass grafts (often veins) respond well to stents.

Medication After the Procedure. After angioplasty with a stent, an anticoagulant such as Coumadin will be prescribed daily for two months, as well as aspirin, another anticlotting medication called Persantine, and a calcium channel blocker such as Cardizem or Procardia.

Directional and Rotational Coronary Atherectomy and Laser Angioplasty

Because medical science is always looking for a newer, better method of opening narrowed arteries, other nonsurgical techniques have been pioneered. *Directional coronary atherectomy* uses a cutting tool mounted on a catheter to shave the plaque off the blood vessel. This device moves back and forth in the vessel, slicing off the deposits. *Rotational atherectomy* uses a tiny rotating tip, covered with thousands of microscopic diamond crystals, to whirr through the plaque. It breaks the blockage into tiny particles, even smaller than a red blood cell. The natural action of the body allows these particles to be absorbed into the bloodstream as they are washed away. Some devices have a collection chamber for storing the plaque as it breaks apart. The plaque is removed when the catheter is withdrawn. The procedure is usually repeated several times to get as much plaque out as possible.

These treatments take about as long as an angioplasty and have the same recovery time. Some studies credit atherectomy with an 85 percent success rate. However, there is still an incidence of vessel closure, which necessitates an immediate bypass. And as you may imagine in a procedure where cutting is done inside a very small area, there are many complications. None of the data show that healing is significantly better than with angioplasty.

Laser angioplasty is now being used in clinical trials. In this procedure, a laser tip is introduced with the balloon. As the balloon inflates and rips up the edges of the plaque, the laser tacks down the edges of tissue. Supposedly the procedure offers better healing than either traditional angioplasty or directional atherectomy. But it is really too soon to say what the long-term benefits of this procedure will be. Currently, this procedure is more commonly used for peripheral vascular disease, to treat blockages in the leg.

What You Need to Know About Open Heart Surgery

When the coronary arteries are massively blocked or narrowed and angioplasty is either unsuccessful, or repeated angioplasties have failed to keep them open, you may have to consider open heart surgery. The New York Heart Association Patient

Classification for potential candidates suggests that patients should have an obstruction greater than 70 percent of the diameter of the affected artery and have chronic angina that hasn't responded to medical or noninvasive treatment. Unstable angina—the type that gives pain even when you aren't exerting yourself—is also an indication for this operation.

The operation, known as CABG (coronary artery bypass grafting), was first pioneered in the 1960s, and it has certainly come a very long way since then. Although the operation is far more commonly performed on men, today women who have already undergone catheterization have just about an equal chance of being referred for bypass surgery as their male counterparts.

This is by no means an experimental treatment anymore; 407,000 were performed in 1991 alone—only one quarter of them on women and nearly half on individuals under the age of sixty-five. CABG is major surgery, and the complications and risks are formidable. However, if you qualify as a candidate for this procedure, it could not only save your life but also improve the quality of your life.

What Does Bypass Entail? If you think of the way that cars can become backed up on a busy thoroughfare, you can imagine the problems that arise in the "highways" that carry blood to your heart. But just as mechanical engineers can build overpasses and detours around highway obstruction, so surgeons can reroute blood flow from diseased and narrowed arteries into new channels created from a vein or artery taken from somewhere else in the body.

Surgeons generally use a vein from the leg or the mammary artery from the chest as their bypass graft. Most people interviewed said that surprisingly the healing process was most difficult and painful when the graft was taken from the leg, which can be swollen and tender for weeks or even months. The mammary artery from the chest wall, on the other hand, tends to stay open longer, although this graft can be more difficult to use. Cosmetically, it's not as pleasing. The scar from bypass surgery runs through the middle of your breastbone with two other

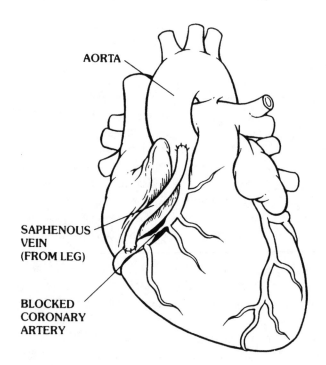

AORTA

SAPHENOUS
VEIN
(FROM LEG)

BLOCKED
CORONARY
ARTERY

**CORONARY BYPASS USING THE SAPHENOUS VEIN
(FROM LEG)**

Reproduced with permission.
"Answers by Heart Patient Information Sheets," 1994
Copyright © American Heart Association.

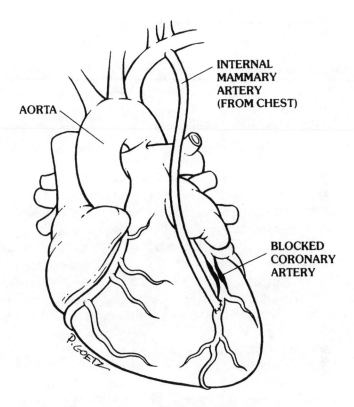

**CORONARY BYPASS USING THE INTERNAL
MAMMARY ARTERY (FROM CHEST)**

puncture scars beneath that from the drains that are placed in the body during surgery. But the graft taken from your leg also involves a scar down the length of your leg.

You don't need to worry about losing any function once the vein or artery is moved. The body has other arteries and can get along fine when just one or two have been moved to the heart. The other leg veins take over the function of the one that has been removed.

What Are the Risks for Women? Unfortunately, the mortality rate for women undergoing this procedure is almost twice that of men—about 4.6 percent for women and 2.6 percent for men, according to a 1987 study. There are no significant current studies to indicate that the percentage has changed, although improved surgical equipment and techniques have probably improved women's prognosis in general.

Of course, these statistics reflect surgery on individuals who are usually older and sicker when they are recommended for this intensive surgical procedure. In a postmenopausal woman, the veins and arteries are less elastic than they are in younger women. And some of the higher death rate is attributable to the occasional increase in postoperative heart failure in women because of diastolic dysfunction.

The positives and negatives of the surgical outcome aren't just determined by gender, however—the more severe the extent of the disease and the higher the number of additional medical illnesses, the greater the risk of death, whether you're a woman or a man. And of course these statistics also reflect delayed treatment in women who should have gotten more aggressive therapies sooner.

When we look at the long-term survival rates, the picture is brighter for women. Both the Coronary Artery Surgery Study (CASS) of 1984 and the more recent MITI Registry data show that if women live six months past their bypass, they do quite well. Although about 13 percent of women die in the hospital or after the procedure, as opposed to 6.5 percent of men, the five- and ten-year survival rates are about the same. Past that time, however, the outcomes are not as good. According to the Office of Women's Health at the National Institutes of Health, only 46 percent of women who have bypass surgery survive for twelve years, as compared with 61 percent of men who have the procedure.

But when you're looking at these numbers, take into consideration the fact that a seventy-year-old woman simply has a shorter life expectancy than a forty-year-old man—regardless of what kind of surgery she undergoes. And twelve years later, her life expectancy is considerably shorter.

This operation is not a "cure" for coronary artery disease. Although the wonders of surgical science can open a clogged artery, it will only *stay* open if the individual drastically changes her lifestyle. Returning to a sedentary, stressful life, smoking cigarettes and eating a high-fat diet will assuredly damage the arteries and the new bypass. So you must be dedicated and motivated to change if you wish to undergo this difficult, expensive, and risky procedure.

Are You a Good Candidate for Open Heart Surgery?

A woman who meets the following criteria is a good candidate for heart surgery. She:

- Has blockage in at least two coronary arteries
- Has blockage in her left main artery
- Is otherwise healthy (no kidney disease, diabetes, etc.)
- Has good heart muscle function (that is, no heart failure)
- Is under seventy-five
- Has a positive attitude about the outcome of the procedure.

You are *higher risk* if:

- You have already suffered a heart attack
- You have other medical problems, such as diabetes or kidney disease

- You have several different forms of heart disease (coronary artery disease and a valve problem, for example)
- This is an emergency procedure
- You are over seventy-five.

And so the question remains, should you venture into the potentially dangerous waters of bypass surgery? Each case, of course, is individual. However, if the quality of your life is severely impaired by chest pain, shortness of breath, and chronic fatigue, or if your physician has told you that you will not be able to live out a full life without surgery, then you may feel that the considerable risks are worth a new chance at life. These are questions to be pondered with your family and friends, with your physician, and alone, in the privacy of your heart.

How to Pick a Hospital. The place where your open heart surgery is performed can make the difference between life and death. If you are a very high risk candidate, you should seriously consider the dedicated heart centers—the Cleveland Clinic in Ohio, the Washington Hospital Center in Washington, DC, the Mayo Clinic in Minnesota, and Massachusetts General Hospital in Boston are the most highly regarded in the country.

If you are moderate to low risk, there are many other facilities that will serve you well. You may wish to be at a teaching hospital, where cutting-edge medicine is being practiced, and you are the patient of a team that includes new, sharp minds and hands. Or you may decide against a teaching hospital, since generally you will see not the prestigious primary surgeon but the second-string players, who have less experience and work under the "star."

Or you may select a hospital on the basis of your cardiologist's recommendation for a cardiac surgeon. If you have found a doctor you trust who has an excellent reputation for success in this operation, he or she is probably affiliated with an excellent institution.

Find out how many cardiac procedures are performed annually

at the hospital you're considering (the number should be at least 250), and request information (yours for the asking!) about their morbidity and mortality rates (complications and death rates).

Your Team: The Medical Professionals

You begin with your *internist*, the physician who is responsible for your general health and can refer you to specialists along the way. If she has noted anything unusual about your heart in a regular physical exam, she will refer you to a cardiologist.

The *cardiologist* is the physician who will ultimately make the decision to refer you for surgery after she has tried medication and noninvasive procedures to treat your heart disease. This individual is responsible for making your diagnosis, ordering the various tests that will determine your condition, and recommending you for surgery.

Your cardiologist will refer you to a *cardiac* or *cardiovascular surgeon*, who is going to be the team leader on your surgical case.

Surgical assistants (some will be residents in a teaching facility) coordinate your in-hospital examinations and testing and will assist at the operation.

The *anesthesiologist* is responsible for keeping you in a deep state of unconsciousness throughout the operation. The night before your surgery, he will come to your room and interview you about your allergies and the medications you take, as well as asking about any adverse effects you've had to anesthesia in the past. He'll be responsible for monitoring your vital signs and giving the fluids and medications you will need while the operation progresses.

The *perfusionist* on the heart-lung machine will coordinate with the surgeons and the anesthesiologist to make sure that your circulation and respiration are maintained mechanically throughout the operation.

The *scrub nurses* will provide expert assistance throughout the procedure and are specially trained in operating room techniques.

As you wake up, the *surgical intensive care nurses* will be at your side to monitor your progress. They will be on duty around the clock to check your vital signs and be sure that you are recovering well from surgery.

What to Do Prior to Surgery

- Read as much as you can about this procedure.
- Consider donating a few pints of your own blood. You usually do not need a transfusion during open heart surgery, but if complications should arise, you want to know that the blood supplied to you is absolutely safe. Your own blood is the best solution, and you can ask friends and family who have the same blood type to donate as well. Screening procedures for hepatitis and the HIV virus since 1985 are vastly improved, thanks to the vigilance of the American Red Cross, but there are occasional horror stories. So by taking charge of this part of your surgery, you are one step ahead.
- Find out from your doctor which medications might be contraindicated right before your surgery and stop taking them.
- Make provisions at work and at home for someone to take over for you while you recuperate.
- Join a support group, or find one to join while you recuperate.
- Ask questions of all your medical professionals! During your preoperative appointments, and at any time up to and including the morning of your surgery, be sure to address all your concerns. The following list may help you become a more informed and more confident patient.

QUESTIONS TO ASK YOUR DOCTOR BEFORE SURGERY
- Is this surgery absolutely necessary? Why?
- Is there another medication we can try before resorting to surgery? Or a different dosage of the medication I'm currently on?

- Is there any other less risky procedure that might yield the same or similar results as an operation?
- Will you agree to do the surgery after I've had a second opinion by another physician of my choice?
- Where will my incision be? How long will it be?
- Do you plan to take a vein from my leg as opposed to my mammary artery? How long will the leg take to heal? How unsightly will this be in stockings?
- What does the surgery entail? (If you're not sure of where your organs are, ask to see a model or drawing.)
- What are the risks of this surgery?
- What are the risks of the anesthesia I'll be given, and are there any side effects?
- Do you think I should have blood drawn before surgery in case I need a transfusion?
- How long will I be in the hospital?
- When can I expect to see you in the hospital?
- When can I shower or bathe?
- What is your fee for surgery? What are the other costs I'll incur? (Hospital stay, anesthesiologist's fee, etc.)

WHAT HAPPENS AFTER THE SURGERY?
- Should I stay in bed when I get home, and for how long?
- What are the warning signs of infection that I should be alert to?
- What are your instructions on nutrition and exercise?
- What are my restrictions on activity and lifting?
- When can I return to work?
- Will I be interested in sex?
- How do I get over my terror of endangering my health if I have an orgasm? How do I talk to my partner about getting back to sexuality slowly together?
- Are there any special instructions my partner and I should have about positions and sexual behaviors?
- What if I feel very depressed? What should I do?

- Could there be a recurrence of my condition? When? How will I know that the bypass was not successful in treating my heart disease?
- When should I schedule a follow-up visit with you?

What Is the Preoperative Procedure?

Before your operation, you'll have some tests that you've undoubtedly had before. However, they must be repeated in order to give your cardiac surgeon the most up-to-date information about you and your heart. You will have:

- an ECG
- a chest X ray
- laboratory work (blood and urine)
- the night before surgery, your leg may be shaved if the surgeon intends to take a vein. It is easier to scrub skin and get it sterile if there is no hair on it.

How Is the Operation Performed?

You will be given a Valium or similar medication in your room to relax you before you are taken to the ER. In a holding room outside the operating room, the anesthesiologist will place an intravenous line in your arm for initial sedation, and you will be brought into the OR. He'll place an oxygen line in your nose and will then intubate you (place a tube down your throat) so that you can be connected to a machine that will regulate your breathing.

Through the IV, you'll be given various medications and narcotics to keep you deeply asleep. You will also have a catheter in your wrist to monitor your arterial blood pressure and one in your jugular vein threaded through to your heart to monitor blood pressure. Throughout the procedure, samples of your blood and urine will be taken to the laboratory and results will be called into the operating room.

The surgeon will begin by cutting through your breastbone to open the chest and expose your beating heart. He will put tubing in place that will connect up with the heart-lung machine so that a smooth transfer can be made before he starts his graft. Because your blood will be rerouted temporarily through the machine, very little blood is lost in the process.

Your body temperature will be lowered to between 24 and 35 degrees centigrade (77 to 88 degrees Fahrenheit), in order to slow the pace of the beating heart and to cut back on the heart's requirement for oxygenated blood. The perfusionist and anesthesiologist will then be alerted that it is time to switch you over to the heart-lung machine. The anesthesiologist will give you an anticoagulant such as Heparin to prevent your blood from clotting while you are on the heart-lung machine.

Then the surgeon will clamp your aorta and apply an infusion of saline and cold water, stopping your heart. Your circulation will then continue through the tubing in your heart to the heart-lung machine.

One of the surgical assistants will then remove either the saphenous vein from your leg or your mammary artery to begin the graft. One opening is made in the aorta and another below the blockage in the damaged artery. An end of the vein or artery used for the bypass is sewn to each end and a new route is then created for blood flow. The graft takes over for the piece of coronary artery that can no longer fulfill its function. Evidently, if you have blockages in more than one artery, this procedure must be repeated for each bypass.

Next, you and your circulatory system must be reunited. The anesthesiologist and perfusionist will work together to bring your temperature back up and slowly wean you off the heart-lung machine. As warm blood reaches the heart, it begins pumping again on its own, although sometimes arrhythmias may set in. The surgeon may apply an electric shock with a defibrillator to get your heartbeat back on track. When he's satisfied with your heart's restored rhythm, he and his colleagues will close your chest with stainless steel wires, and the anesthesiologist will deliver another drug, Protamine, to your system, which will neutralize the effect of the Heparin and allow your blood to clot again. Finally, you will be sent to the intensive care unit to recover.

Most open heart procedures take approximately two to three hours, but they can be longer if there are complications.

Recovery in Intensive Care. The worst part is awakening with a tube down your throat, feeling that you're being suffocated. A nurse will be there to calm you and explain how to regulate your breathing so that you can work with the machine. Your vital signs will be monitored here for several hours. If you're doing well, you'll then be transferred to a regular room.

Recovery in an Intermediate Care Unit. For the next few days after surgery, you'll be asked to cough and to puff into a small plastic breathing apparatus every half hour or so. This is called "incentive spirometry" and is essential for clearing secretions from your lungs and windpipe. It is important to keep your lungs in good working order so as to avoid pneumonia, which can be a deadly postsurgical complication.

You will feel most of your pain in your leg, if the graft was taken from there. You'll have an elastic stocking over it to keep the swelling down, but walking may be difficult for the first week or so.

Your chest will be sore, and it may be difficult for you to change position or take deep breaths. You'll be given painkillers and antibiotics to stave off any infection.

How Long Will It Take Until I'm Back to Normal? Recuperation may take several weeks, and you may need three months to feel yourself again. Women may experience depression, sexual dysfunction, and neurological problems after a bypass. It is suspected that some of the impairment that takes place after surgery may have to do with the lessened amount of oxygen the brain gets when you're on the heart-lung machine. It is also possible that small clots could form during surgery that might cause ministrokes—which would of course affect neurological function.

Women, so often the caregivers in their family, must make some adjustments in order to be able to receive care from others while they're getting better. This takes a real change of heart. But if you allow others to do for you as you have done for them (see Chapter 11), you will definitely heal faster and better.

Valve Repair and Replacement

Heart valve replacement surgery is the second most common type of open heart surgery in adults. If you have serious congenital valve problems, or if rheumatic fever or bacterial endocarditis (an infection of the heart) has impaired the function of your valves, you may be recommended for this surgery. The aging process itself may weaken an already overworked valve, requiring repair or a replacement.

When valves stop working properly they either leak and don't close completely (insufficiency or regurgitation), or they stiffen up and can no longer open widely (mitral or aortic stenosis). You may recall from Chapter 2 that the valves are responsible for making sure your blood flows in the right direction from one chamber to another.

Both stenosis and leakage put an increased load on the heart muscle, causing it to become abnormally large. If they occur in more than one valve, or if both conditions occur in the same valve, evidently the burden on the heart is heavier. The resulting symptoms might be difficulty in breathing, fainting, arrhythmias, chest pain, chronic fatigue, or swollen ankles. A bad valve also predisposes you to getting an infection of the heart, which can lead to the formation of blood clots that might trigger a heart attack or a stroke.

Alternatives to Surgery: Balloon Valvuloplasty. Just as angioplasty can open a stenotic artery, so valvuloplasty can be used to widen a stiff valve. The procedures are very similar—a catheter with a balloon tip is run from your femoral artery to the affected valve and then inflated. This technique works best on valves that are not completely stiff and do not have a second complication of leaking.

Advantages of Repairing the Valve. It is, of course,

preferable to keep you own body's organs and tissues rather than replace them. Blood clots are much less common after surgery, and if the operation is successful, your valve has greater longevity than the animal or mechanical replacement valves that are generally used. Your doctor will probably be able to tell from the results of an echocardiogram whether you are a good candidate for repair, although occasionally she will have to defer her opinion until you are already on the operating table.

Valve Repair and Valve Replacement. Both of these procedures require open heart surgery, just like the CABG operation. If you have a leaky mitral valve, it is possible that repair will be recommended, rather than replacement. A leaky aortic valve is a much more difficult job to repair, so replacement may be the best course of action.

If the valve is damaged beyond repair, it is removed and then replaced by either a long-lasting mechanical valve, made of metal and plastic, or a tissue valve usually taken from a pig, which is the animal whose heart is closest to the human model.

The mechanical valve is extremely durable, but if you have one, you must take Coumadin, a blood thinner, for the rest of your life. This is a powerful medication which can prolong bleeding and requires you to be subjected to regular blood tests and careful monitoring of the dosage of your medication.

The advantage of the tissue valve from the pig is that it doesn't require a blood thinner. The disadvantage, however, is that this replacement doesn't last as long as the mechanical variety. Just like the parts of a human heart, an animal valve undergoes wear and damage over time.

How Is the Procedure Performed? The course of the operation follows that of open heart surgery—you are put on a heart-lung machine, and the surgeon then opens the pericardium, cutting through the atrium or aorta to get to the damaged valve. If he cannot repair it, he removes it and places the new valve between the chambers, sewing it into place. When the heart is closed, you are weaned off the heart-lung machine and your heart takes over again. You may wish to bank your blood, in case it is needed during the surgery.

After valve replacement, it is absolutely essential that you keep your new valve healthy. Because it is a foreign body, it is a good target for infections of the heart (bacterial endocarditis). This means you must follow your doctor's instructions to the letter when he prescribes antibiotics for infections, and even preventively, before dental or surgical procedures.

Helping Your Mind to Heal Your Body

We know that we can benefit greatly from allowing the mind to heal the body—even as we require high-tech procedures such as open heart surgery and valvuloplasty. If you've been staying healthy with heart disease but have arrived at a point where you've completed all the physical steps—from medication to noninvasive treatment to bypass or valve surgery—it is time to tackle the more elusive emotional and spiritual issues. Chapter 11 will offer you new ways to look at your old life—and offer options for goal planning, lifestyle modification, sexual vitality, and peace of mind.

But it is also true that the heart has crises that we cannot prevent. As much as we may attempt to stave off the ravages of a heart attack, it does occur and can disrupt the best healing program. It is vital to know when you are in crisis and exactly what to do about it. The next chapter will take you along the difficult journey from heart attack to recovery.

10

Surviving a Heart Attack
▽

It is terrifying and overwhelming; or we don't even know it has occurred. It is crushing and painful, or silent and deadly. This is the beast known as a heart attack.

What exactly is a myocardial infarction? We have to recognize it in order to deal with it. The amazing thing is that many women refuse to admit that this traumatic cardiac event is taking place—often, not until it is too late.

We need to know exactly what a heart attack looks like, what you might feel when you're going through it, and what might happen to you as you are rushed to the hospital and into treatment. Only then will you be able to meet the beast head-on and fight it with all the resources available to you.

What Is a Heart Attack?

A heart attack is the end point of years of arterial plaque blocking arteries and of blood vessels constricting. The final blow is usually the rupture of a plaque and the complete loss of blood flow to a region of the heart. When blood does not move through the arteries, oxygen is not present either, and this can severely damage the heart muscle. There may be a blockage in one or more of the coronary arteries, which feed blood to the heart muscle, or a plaque may have ruptured, forming a blood clot. We have all seen the public service announcements dramatizing the classic male heart attack: the man is sitting in an easy chair watching television. He feels uneasy and shifts in his chair, then abruptly gets up and yells to his daughter in the next room to stop making so much noise. As he eases himself back into the chair, we see a look of horror cross his face. He grips his left arm and can't seem to get a breath. He breaks out in a sweat and can't even raise his arm to loosen his tie. When his wife walks into the room, he appears dazed. He stares blindly into space, unable even to accept her concern.

Will this same scene happen to a woman? It might, but then again, it might not. Typically, women suffer angina—or chest pain—for years, whereas men more often have an acute myocardial infarction (heart attack) as their first symptom. But an initial infarction for a woman is more likely to be fatal. In the Framingham Heart Study, 39 percent of deaths in women occurred when they had a heart attack as a first symptom, as opposed to 31 percent in men.

Claudia, a thirty-eight-year-old civilian paramedic, a lieutenant in the fire department, refused to believe that the pain she was experiencing was a heart attack—even though she'd witnessed countless dozens of similar experiences in other men and women in the course of her work. But when it hit home, it hit too close. All she wanted to do was ignore it—and go back to work.

"I knew it was ridiculous," she said. "I had work to do. People depended on me for their lives! I handled all our bills, our taxes, all the major decisions. I'd fought to get custody of my niece when my sister was killed in a car crash. I mean, look at all this evidence that I was in charge of my life—it was totally impossible that I was having a heart attack."

Claudia didn't report until the very end of our interview that she was a heavy smoker, but the tension coming out of her was palpable. She was angry at her body, angry that she couldn't perform as a mother and a paramedic when she was sick, angry at her supervisors for trying to take away her job after her crisis. She felt out of control, as if she had no way to reconcile the fact that she'd put her heart and soul into her job and her heart had betrayed her, big time.

Claudia's daily life was shift work—twenty-four hours on, seventy-two hours off—which meant that she had to find exceptional baby-sitters who would work literally round the clock to take care of Lucy, who was four weeks old. Then she had to keep herself in good shape so that she could be superwoman—paramedic, mother, wife. Every three years, the department required a physical, so she knew her cholesterol was fine, though her blood pressure was high enough to require a diuretic, Maxide. On her own, she started taking niacin and an aspirin a day. Her doctor strongly suggested that she enter a smoking-cessation program, but she didn't have time for that.

The following Halloween, she got the scare of her life. She was scheduled to take a management class to help prepare her for a promotion in the fire department hierarchy. She climbed the flight of stairs to the classroom and was nearly thrown back down them by the violent pain in her chest.

"Just like every patient I've ever had," she said. "There it was—the elephant sitting right on me. I wanted to scream but I couldn't make a sound. My pal, also a paramedic, saw me clutch at my chest, and he reached over to take my pulse. But somehow, I was still standing on my feet, and I convinced myself that it wasn't so bad. My friend said my pulse was fast, that I was probably nervous about taking this class.

"So I went into the room and took my seat and took notes. By lunchtime, the pain had subsided. I had a bowl of soup and some salad and we went back to the office building and climbed those damn stairs again. And it happened again. So what, I thought, I ate too fast.

"That night, I took my daughter trick or treating, and went to sleep. But the next day, I couldn't get out of bed. I slept in till about noon and then got up and started sorting laundry. I was really angry at my husband—I think he'd thrown some colored sheets in with the whites—something dumb like that. Then I wasn't angry anymore because I was hit by the chest pain again, and this time, I understood. It was the big one. I realized I didn't have much time left.

"I didn't call 911—I *work* 911, and I know better. I called a neighbor and told her to get me to the hospital. It was crazy, she kept apologizing for the broken seat belt and the fact that her husband kept meaning to get new brakes. I just kept counting minutes. How long did I have before the damage was complete? How long did I have to live?

"We got there, and I think it was fifteen minutes total from when the pain hit. I was so hot, burning up. I tried to move to get away from the pain, but I didn't have the strength. They got me out of the car and all I could say as they stuck me on a gurney was, 'Get my pants off, I'm too hot.' "

The nurse got a line started and they drew blood to check Claudia's enzymes. They asked a million questions—when was her last menstrual period, what medications was she on, had she eaten recently? The emergency room doctor ordered tPA (transplasminogen activator), but made her sign a release. Later, Claudia learned that all the fuss about this medication was justified—the doctor had made a radical choice in selecting this new type of thrombolytic therapy because he worried that, as a young woman in her reproductive years who still had menstrual periods, the tPA might trigger uncontrollable bleeding. But in fact the tPA saved her life.

How Do You Know This Is "The Big One"?

Claudia's situation is all too common. Women refuse to acknowledge that this major event has taken place. Because if they admit to the heart attack, they admit to their own vulnerability.

It is crucial, first, to know what you might feel if in fact you are hit by a heart attack. Some symptoms that women experience during an attack may be different from those that men experience:

- a heavy fullness or pressure like chest pain between breasts and radiating to left arm or shoulder
- weakness and lethargy
- nausea
- clammy perspiration (*diaphoresis*)
- shortness of breath
- pain traveling down left or right arm
- angina felt as back pain or deep aching and throbbing in left or right bicep or forearm
- a feeling of portending doom—as though some terrible event is about to happen
- or no symptoms at all—the so-called silent heart attack that only registers on a subsequent ECG.

The most important thing that can be said about a heart attack is that **time is of the essence.** If you are at risk and you have any of the above symptoms, or a cluster of them, you should already have an emergency plan set with your physician, family, and friends. **Don't assume it is indigestion or the flu! Don't wait!** The majority of women who have heart attacks remain in denial hours—even days—after the event. And the longer the heart is deprived of oxygen, the more cells die. Certain medications, like clot busters, must be given within six to twelve hours of the onset of the attack to be effective. A severely damaged heart is much more difficult to save than a slightly damaged heart—and if more than six hours have gone by since the attack began without oxygen being restored to the heart, there may be little heart muscle left to salvage.

How Do You Know You're Having a Heart Attack?

Jennifer, whom we met in Chapter 2, described her heart attack as an octopus gripping her chest. No matter what she did—recline her seat, get up, change position—the pain wouldn't stop. It also radiated down her jaw, back, and left arm. She said that she felt really nauseated, like she wanted to throw up but couldn't. At the same time, she was gasping for breath and had a sense that something awful was happening. (Of course the awful thing was that she was having a heart attack!)

Another heart attack victim eloquently described the event in a poem: "Each breath I took was like/Pushing against crushed glass . . . I sat . . . I paced . . . the pain/In my chest raged."

If you've had angina for years, as Jennifer did, you may be hard put to know the difference between your "everyday pain" and the "big one."

But the time period is significant. Angina is usually a brief pain, and it generally stops when you stop whatever activity you've been doing and sit down. The pain of a heart attack, on the other hand, continues and worsens over a period of twenty minutes or more.

If any of the above descriptions of symptoms fit, don't hesitate. Dial 911 and say, "I am having a heart attack." If you aren't, no one will blame you afterward or accuse you of lying. Fully 35 percent of all heart attacks that occur in women aren't noticed by the woman herself. Denial is one of the worst dangers of heart disease, because the longer you wait, the more damage there will be to the heart muscle.

Do not attempt to drive yourself to the hospital under any circumstances. You may feel capable, but once behind the wheel, under the pressure and stress of negotiating traffic, finding your way and being anxious about your condition, you could have an irregular heart rhythm and black out. This could severely jeopardize not only yourself, but also other drivers.

Be Prepared for Emergencies—Make a Plan

Anyone can have a heart attack. Even you. Perhaps, especially you. And the more prepared you can be, the better. If you have already been diagnosed with any form of heart disease, or if you have a strong family history, you should take the time to compile a detailed instruction sheet of information about your health status and your wishes about medical treatment. If you have all your names and phone numbers, medical history, and advance directives for care down in writing, no one can contradict your requests or claim ignorance of your condition. By communicating your needs and wishes, you will get better care when the ambulance arrives and when you are admitted to the emergency room.

The following lists will help you and anyone who might be present when you're having a heart attack. The first is a personal preparation, the second is a list for the triage nurse in the hospital. Compile these carefully, with the help from your doctor, and keep them in a folder next to your phone. Your list for the nurse should travel with you to the hospital in case you are unconscious and can't talk for yourself. When you are wheeled in the emergency room door, the person who brought you in should hand it to the triage nurse.

Getting the Help You Need During a Heart Attack

FOR YOURSELF

1. Keep your physician's number and all numbers of close friends and relatives by the phone.

2. Understand how 911 works and use it to your advantage. In most cities, large hospitals have a hookup between 911 and their MICU (mobile intensive care unit). Any individual having a heart attack can call the emergency line and expect an intensive care unit on wheels within minutes. Many of them carry ACLS (advanced cardiac life-support) providers and their equipment. In some areas, an operator will stay on the line with you or the caller who dialed 911 and explain exactly what to do until the unit arrives.

3. If you own a computer with a modem and have access to E-mail transmissions, your quickest response, and the one you might be most capable of if you're in pain, may be to type in a message to other members of the electronic network who will be

on-line at the time. In cities or rural areas where 911 response may not be immediate, and the chances are fifty-fifty that you'll get an answering machine when you make a phone call to a close friend or relative, the computer can be a lifeline.

4. If you are fortunate enough to be with another person when a heart attack strikes, and your heart stops, your companion should begin CPR (cardiopulmonary resuscitation) immediately. The quicker oxygen can be restored to the heart and brain, the better the chance that there will be little or no cardiac or brain damage. Even an untrained person can do chest compressions and mouth-to-mouth breathing until the ambulance arrives and the paramedics can take over. Your companion must keep going no matter how long or how futile it seems. Once CPR has begun, it cannot be terminated until a doctor has pronounced the patient dead.

5. If you are conscious, you must be your own advocate in the emergency room and make sure your companion backs you up. Many women are too exhausted to be assertive, and too polite to violate the "last in, last served" rule. Don't ever wait for care, even if the place is jam-packed. Tell the triage nurse, who decides the order of patients to be treated, that you are having a heart attack and must be attended to immediately.

FOR THE HOSPITAL STAFF

1. Make a written plan, with the help of your physician, for what might happen if you should have a heart attack. This plan should include a decision about administering thrombolytic drugs based on whether or not you have any history of unusual bleeding. Your plan should also have the name of the cardiac surgeon recommended by your doctor, should you need open heart surgery.

2. Since all jurisdictions in the United States require that ambulance crews take the patient to the nearest facility, write down the name and number of your personal physician and her hospital affiliation so that she can be contacted immediately if you are in a different hospital.

3. Make sure you have written advance directives and a living will that will authorize your family or friends to make decisions about life-saving treatments if you are unconscious or physically or mentally impaired.

What Drugs and Treatments Will I Get in the Emergency Room?

Things will happen fast in the emergency room—doctors, nurses, and ambulance personnel will be rushing around, caring for you with split-second efficiency. Don't expect any bedside manner—in the interests of saving time, no one will pay much attention to treating you like an individual or will even ask how you're feeling. The attending staff want to make sure they get your body stabilized as quickly as they can.

INITIAL EXAMINATION

When you are admitted to the emergency room, the on-duty physician will take your *pulse* and *blood pressure*. He will take a *history* and question you about the nature of the pain you're experiencing—when it started, where it is located, how long it has persisted, whether it ebbs and flows or is constant.

You will then have an *ECG* and *blood* will be drawn.

Blood work. There are special enzymes that appear in the blood several hours after an attack, emitted by the dying heart cells. These enzymes, abbreviated as CPK, CK-MB, and LDH, remain detectable for three or four days. If your test is positive for these enzymes, they will confirm your physician's suspicion that you have suffered a heart attack.

MEDICATIONS

1. Nitroglycerin. This will be administered to dilate the blood vessels—it may also alleviate the pain in your chest as your blood flow improves.

2. Antiarrhythmic drugs. Lidocaine will be administered if you are experiencing certain arrhythmias. This drug will restore the heart's rhythm to normal. If your heart rhythm becomes very abnormal (a condition known as *ventricular tachycardia*) you may be stimulated with electric paddles to shock the heart back to a normal rhythm.

3. Diuretics. The physician will probably order a diuretic to remove fluid from the body. **Lasix** or **Bumex** may be administered if you are having difficulty breathing, and the admitting doctor can hear fluid in the lungs. This can be a sign of congestive heart failure. (See Chapter 9 for a full description of these drugs.)

4. Antihypertensive drugs. It is important to reduce blood pressure after a heart attack (just the anxiety of your trip in the ambulance might have raised your pressure abnormally). There are several varieties of drugs given, including *beta-blockers, calcium channel blockers,* and *ACE inhibitors* (see Chapter 9 for a full explanation of these drugs and how they work).

5. Thrombolytic drugs. The drugs in this category, known as "clot busters," actually break up the clots in your arteries. They can be lifesavers, but they can also be risky. If you have any history of abnormal bleeding, a recent major surgery, or a recent stroke, thrombolysis may not be for you. Also, in order for a doctor to consider administering these drugs, the physician must see abnormalities on your ECG. Clot busters work best if administered within six hours after the heart attack, although they can be given up to twelve hours after chest pain began.

Streptokinase, which is effective for about three hours, had been the drug of choice until **tPA (transplasminogen activator),** a genetically engineered enzyme, was developed in a laboratory. Patients who received streptokinase in a timely fashion had up to 47 percent fewer deaths than those who didn't get the therapy. Blockage was dissolved in 40 to 80 percent of the cases.

6. Painkillers. If you are in pain, you will also be given **morphine.** A great deal of controversy has arisen over the ramifications of not alleviating pain sufficiently. Morphine and its derivatives are only addictive when administered over a long time in increasing dosages. If pain relief is given *before* severe pain sets in, a lower dosage will do the job. Morphine also helps lower blood pressure and improves the shortness of breath associated with a heart attack. The other benefit of this narcotic is that it can help to remove the awful sense of doom and anxiety typically experienced by a person having a heart attack.

Make sure that you don't suffer in silence. If you are in so much discomfort that you can't relax, you are under undue stress and may cause your heart more damage.

POSSIBLE EMERGENCY TREATMENTS

1. Catheterization. A cardiologist may decide to catheterize you at this time, in order to determine the extent of blockage in your arteries. The results will determine whether or not you should have an angioplasty immediately to open the blocked artery. (See Chapter 8 for a description of this procedure.)

2. Angioplasty. If the catheterization shows definite blockage, the physician may decide to do an angioplasty to open the artery. (See Chapter 9 for a description of this procedure.) But if the balloon catheter is not able to pass across the blockage, and the heart is in danger of dying from lack of oxygen, your cardiologist may opt for an emergency bypass operation.

3. Emergency Bypass Surgery. The bypass operation, described in Chapter 9, has allowed thousands of individuals to survive heart attacks. Procedures performed during an emergency are of necessity done under pressure, so this is something you must discuss seriously with your doctor when you are well. Your medical plan should include contingencies for every occurrence, and it will alleviate a certain amount of your anxiety to know all about the bypass operation before you are rushed into surgery.

Do Women Receive Equal Treatment in the Emergency Room?

Are women treated less carefully than men or taken less seriously if they come to the emergency room with a heart attack? This all depends on the personnel on duty at the time. It has been documented that there are still emergency room staff who pay less attention to a woman admitted for a heart attack than a man. Grace, whom we met in Chapter 7, had to come back to the emergency room—not once but three times—when she swore she was having an attack. On the other hand, Katharine, who told us her story in Chapter 3, was told immediately by the doctor on duty that she was a classic case, and they were sending her right up to the intensive care unit.

A study performed on 4,891 patients in Seattle, Washington, who were admitted to hospitals for heart attacks, showed that women were not treated the same as men—they were less likely to be given clot busters, to be catheterized, or to be given balloon angioplasty. Another study, from the Office of Women's Health, showed that women who had heart attacks remained in local hospitals an average of 4.5 days before being transferred to a larger hospital for more advanced treatment, though men were transferred after 2.4 days. But a more recent 1992 study from Beth Israel Hospital in Boston on about half as many patients showed that men and women did get relatively equal treatment. It is possible that as more physicians become more aware that women's heart disease is every bit as dangerous and worthy of treatment as men's, new studies will show a balance in medical care.

If you are given a perfunctory exam without adequate attention being paid to your description of the event, the on-call doctor may decide to discharge you. If you feel in any way uncomfortable about this, you should refuse to sign the discharge papers and request a cardiologist for a second opinion. You should also ask the staff to notify your personal physician so that you can discuss your options with her.

What Goes on During Your Hospital Stay?

You will be transferred from the emergency room to the CCU (coronary care unit) for the next twenty-four to thirty-six hours. During that time, every breath, every heartbeat will be watched and recorded. Women are twice as likely as men to die after their first heart attack, so this time is a vital one in terms of healing.

During these critical hours, the doctors will be medicating you to get your heart rhythm back to normal and to alleviate your pain. Medications will range from painkillers and nitroglycerin to medications to make your heart beat more strongly to blood pressure medication—beta-blockers or ACE inhibitors (see Chapter 9). Your blood pressure will be monitored, often by a catheter inserted in an artery, and an ECG monitor will run continuously.

As soon as your condition and vital signs are stable, you will be transferred to a regular floor, although some hospitals have cardiac "step-down units" as an intermediary stage of recovery. In this unit, usually placed right next to the CCU, you are still monitored continuously, but you are able to get out of bed. The doctors want you up and walking the halls within twenty-four to forty-eight hours after your heart attack if there are no complications. You can eat and go to the bathroom on your own, although a nurse will be present to help you bathe.

Don't Blame Yourself

It is amazing how many people end up in the emergency room lying on the table saying, "I really did it this time." Particularly for women, who are quick to criticize themselves, this punishing reaction can be terribly self-destructive. Are you responsible, in the long run, for your heart attack?

You are, and you aren't. Those who immediately blame the personality—the "type A" excuse—are neglecting so many other factors, such as family history and lipid and hormone levels. On the other hand, those who won't admit that there's any connection between the individual and her illness are also missing a good deal. Certain individuals react so poorly to the tension and anxiety in their lives, they produce an overabundance of stress hormones, which can certainly predispose them to a heart attack.

But it will only do you harm to spend time agonizing over how you might have prevented your cardiac event. What has happened has passed, and you can only deal with the present moment. You may have been a likely candidate to succumb to coronary blockages yesterday, but if you can, try to look at life differently today. Of course you aren't going to become a different person overnight, but there's no reason to assume you'd want to repeat your recent traumatic experience. Give yourself the benefit of the doubt—you're here not to blame yourself but to heal yourself.

Nothing to Fear But Fear of the Heart Attack Itself

It is terrifying to experience a heart attack, but it is far more dangerous to ignore the attack or claim it is not happening than to look the creature in the eyes and deal with it. The quicker you respond to what's happening in your body, the better your chances of preventing serious damage to your heart.

Having a heart attack is an experience that shakes us to our very roots. But we can come out on the other side, wiser and healthier than before. In the next chapter, we'll talk about the road back. It may be long and hard, but the destination is well worth it.

11

Recuperation and Recovery:
How to Prevent a Second Attack

▽

After a heart attack, you may be fragile and vulnerable; you may be desperate to recapture your life as it was before. Or you may feel that this is a true beginning, a chance to start over. After all, for the health of your heart, you have to make some significant additions and subtractions from the life you used to live. Whatever your reaction to surviving a heart attack—fear, hope, relief, or a true conviction that this awful event happened in order to wake you up—you have the power to make a real difference in your future.

Mary, who was forty-eight when she had her attack, put it this way: "I was divorced, living on my own. The day it happened, a sunny day in 1980, I was at the beach. The water looked pretty calm, and I waded out into it.

"Then, in the next second, I was down. An undercurrent whipped my legs out from under me. I had no breath left and a tightness right in the center of my chest, and it was impossible for me to get my footing. I was carried out by the tide—I think the only thing that saved me was that I remembered not to wave but to make a fist and punch the air instead. A couple of teenagers spotted me and dragged me out before I went under completely. I was panting like I'd run a race and was out of steam.

"The thing of it was, despite my high blood pressure, which I kept under control with Aldomet, I was not a sick woman. Even when I was coming up for air, I kept thinking, This is wrong, this shouldn't be happening to me. I had a totally nonstressful life—I was a dog groomer—and I'd quit smoking five years earlier. I was thin, ate a good diet, my cholesterol and triglycerides were normal. Sure, there was a family history—an aunt on my mother's side who had died of a heart condition at sixteen, and an aunt on my father's side who died in her forties of another heart condition. My father had died of a heart attack six years before I had mine, when he was sixty-nine. But I'd never thought it could happen to me.

"When I got home, I went to my family doctor and I said, 'I had a heart attack. And I never want to have another one.' He was very sympathetic—he said a good recuperation was the key."

In those days, they put heart patients on complete bed rest in the hospital for two or three weeks. Mary couldn't imagine taking care of herself when she was released. The idea of coming home alone was scary, and she didn't want to burden her mother with her care, so she opted for a rehabilitation hospital for the next two weeks. By the time she was discharged, she was champing at the bit to get back to real life again. And she vowed she was going to keep up the good work of rehabilitating her life.

"It's about fourteen years since my heart attack," Mary said, "and I'm still on blood pressure medication. Through the years, my doctor has been very supportive about how I live. Of course he told me to eat well and keep active and go easy on the coffee. But what really made the difference in my mental and physical health was my marriage to Ted.

"I didn't have enough time with Ted [Mary's husband died of a stroke in 1994], but when he was in my life, he helped to change my whole outlook. I was always running, and he'd say, 'It's all right, take it easy.' I listened to him and started to live more like he did. Now that he's gone, I have my children and friends and I have my practice of the Chinese meditative art, tai chi chuan. I've been doing it for the last two and a half years, and my pressure is now down to 120 over 70. I'm thinking about asking the doctor whether I could try going off medication. I know tai chi has reduced my stress more than anything except Ted.

"I would have to say I do have some limitations since the heart attack. Things are harder for me physically—I still run out of steam and get winded more than I used to. I noticed that my sexual desire wasn't as great since being on the blood pressure pills, but it is hard to tell how much of that was the medicine and how much was lack of energy.

"I never felt sorry for myself through this whole thing. I think it had to do with this one lady at the rehab hospital who always said, 'I'm too sick, I can't do this or that.' She was determined to be an invalid for the rest of her life—well, that wasn't for me! She just confirmed my determination to get well faster."

Getting Back to Work and Play

Mary wisely decided not to go home to care for herself, but instead she chose to spend those important weeks post–heart attack at a rehabilitation hospital. However, if you have a partner, relative, or good friend to stay with you, you can usually go home five to ten days after an attack, or as soon as you're ready to take a modified stress test. You don't need to exercise up to your maximum level to take this test, so don't worry about over-exertion.

You may find it terrifying to be asked to perform any activity that will increase your heart rate. Many women are simply too frightened of bringing on another attack. But the heart—like every other organ in the body—must be used, or we will lose it. Working up to your physical capacity (which may mean working hard emotionally to overcome your fears of bringing on another attack) is the only way to bring you back to normal. Numerous studies have shown that patients who were too fearful of a second attack to get back into the swing of things died with twice the frequency of those who took a deep breath and decided to risk it.

If you do poorly on your exercise stress test before discharge, you haven't "failed" recovery. Rather, this is a good indication to your physician that you may require more than the medication you're on. If this is your case, you may be recommended for cardiac catheterization, to see whether there are any remaining problems, and an echocardiogram, to check the structure and function of the heart muscle.

And if you are recommended for one of these procedures, you will be adding to the numbers of women who are treated "just like a man" after a heart attack—and this is a positive sign. Many doctors forego these tests for their women patients—43 percent of females who had myocardial infarctions underwent procedures to examine or widen narrowed arteries, as opposed to 69 percent of men.

Once your doctor has a good idea of how your heart is healing after the attack and is confident that you are in satisfactory condition, she will ask the social worker at the hospital to come in and discuss the available social services options with you for the next few weeks after you are discharged.

If you have no one to help you at home and need skilled nursing services, she may recommend a rehabilitation hospital (which may not be covered by your insurance plan, and may be difficult to find, depending on where you live), or a home health aide (again, your eligibility depends on your insurance plans and financial situation). Outpatient rehabilitation programs are available from most hospitals, but you will need someone to take you to the site several times a week. Some women who pride themselves on being self-sufficient still find it enormously comforting to know that someone will be coming in several hours a day for the next few weeks to help out.

The hospital staff will give you all sorts of instructions as you check out—from what to eat to how to exercise to what to do in an emergency. Read all pieces of vital information and check them over again during your first week at home. Be sure to call your doctor's office to schedule your post-hospital office visit and also if you have any questions.

Recuperation at Home

When you arrive home, make sure that there is someone to stay with you or check in on you several times a day for the next week. If you are a do-everything person, it will be essential to lie back and allow others to take care of you for a change. This requires an alteration in your expectations for yourself and for others.

Make yourself a schedule for the next few weeks. You need to include meals, naps, showers or baths, time for walking to get back in shape if your doctor has recommended that you exercise, time to write thank-yous for the cards and flowers you undoubtedly got in the hospital, time to sit and think quietly about what you might want to do next.

Make Plans That You Can Accomplish. This is a wonderful opportunity to make short-range plans for doing things you love but rarely do and eliminating things you do regularly that you can't stand.

Consider the Future. Do you really want to continue in the same job you've been doing for years? Is job stress one of the things that landed you in the hospital? If so, think about ways in which you might live differently.

Enlist the Aid of Family and Friends. Many women suffer heart attacks at a time of life when they are living alone, either by choice or because they are widowed or divorced. But for the three to six weeks after your hospitalization, you can't go it alone. If you're not in a rehabilitation hospital or don't have a home health aide coming in, you will need assistance from friends and family. You should investigate all possibilities with the assistance of the social worker at your hospital.

Talk to your closest family members and friends about dividing the work—in most cases, you won't need someone around the clock, but you do need someone to come in several times a day and possibly overnight, depending on your doctor's recommendations.

Get People to Do Things for You. Yes, you're an eminently capable human being. You can probably work your old job from your bed with the help of a fax and phone, you can manage your household, care for a child or grandchild, and write a novel in your spare time. But right now, let other people prove to you how effective they can be in your life. After you've established a support network of friends and family, you have to let them help you. You must believe that things will get done if you delegate them to others to accomplish. They may not get done exactly as you would do them, but is that so terrible? Enjoy letting others surprise you with their style of doing for you.

Call a Nutritionist. You are at a very vulnerable stage when you get out of the hospital, armed with all the menus and meal plans given to you when you were discharged. Because your appetite is probably not yet what it was before your cardiac event, this is a wonderful time to dedicate yourself to new low-fat eating. A nutritionist recommended by your doctor or the American Dietetic Association (see Chapter 13) may set you on a personal course you can live with.

Sign Up for a Rehabilitation Program. Your doctor can recommend a cardiac rehabilitation program and later, a monitored health club program to get your body back in shape.

Take Your Medications As Directed. If you are unused to taking a variety of pills at different times of the day, it may be helpful to keep a log so that you can write down how often to take which pill and what it is for. There are also handy pill dispensers available in drugstores that may help you organize them and remember to take them. Be sure to notify your doctor if you are having any side effects.

See Your Physician. Most cardiologists want to see their patients two weeks after discharge from the hospital. At this time, you can and should discuss more than just how you've been feeling or what effect your medication is having.

Consider Therapy or a Support Group. Isolation is one of the most dangerous risk factors after a heart attack. Women always pride themselves on being able to manage pretty well on their own. But this is the time to gather others close to you and make new attachments to people who can really care—and help. Documented studies show that most individuals can avoid a second heart attack by keeping their blood pressure and cholesterol in check with diet, exercise, and stress management. Your recuperation is the time to consider all the other details that will take you to the threshold of good health and move you over the border, into a new appreciation of life.

Cardiac Rehabilitation—Exercise to Strengthen Your Heart

If your doctor hasn't recommended a cardiac rehabilitation program for you, that's not surprising. Doctors generally recommend such programs to their male patients (who are probably younger and in better shape to begin with) but not so often to females. Why does this bias exist?

In part, it may reflect the typically less aggressive treatment offered to women—but it may also have to do with the doctor/patient relationship. If your physician treats you like a delicate little lady, he is making some assumptions about you that may not be true. If you are seventy-five and rather frail, or if you're overweight and totally sedentary, you may feel as hesitant as your physician about working out. And yet exercise may be what saves you from a second heart attack or bypass.

If the subject of cardiac rehab doesn't come up when you go for your postsurgery or post–heart-attack checkup, you should bring it up. Even if you're out of shape or have never been in shape, even if you haven't sat on a bike since you were a kid, this is the time to start. A study at the Medical Center Hospital of Vermont showed that older women were less likely than older men (15 percent as opposed to 25 percent) to enter a cardiac rehab program and therefore derive the benefits—and you don't want that to happen to you. In this study, those women who did choose to go into the program were in worse shape than the men—at the beginning of the twelve-week course, their peak oxygen consumption was 18 percent lower than the men's. However, after the conditioning program was over, everyone had improved nearly the same amount—peak oxygen consumption had gone up 17 percent in the women and 19 percent in the men. This proves unequivocally that rehabilitation is certainly worthwhile—and you will see the benefits as soon as you start.

A study reported in *Circulation* shows that after a three-month program in endurance training, forty-five patients aged sixty-two to eighty-two who had had a heart attack or bypass increased their capacity for exercise by more than 40 percent.

Two Options for a Rehabilitative Diet Plan After a Heart Attack

Cardiac rehabilitation is an essential portion of your recovery. But if you aren't eating right, the exercise part of your rehabilitation won't mean much. Earlier in this book we outlined a nonrestrictive diet plan, but understand that Chapter 4's regimen is a preventive-care regimen. If you have had a heart attack or bypass surgery, or your cardiac condition is a serious one, you must use more than prevention in order to recover. There are two schools of thought on how you should eat and live to avoid a second cardiac event.

THE ORNISH PLAN

The first school, a plan formulated by Dr. Dean Ornish and practiced by other physicians around the country, is very strict and requires an enormous change of mind and body. It dictates a plant-based, virtually no-fat diet, exceptionally high in complex carbohydrates and low in protein. The regimen prohibits any stimulants that might trigger heart arrhythmias, such as caffeine, nicotine, or recreational drugs, and is almost as restrictive on alcohol. This plan concentrates on diet, but it also mandates daily exercise and daily stress management, which should be an organized program of prayer or meditation to calm the mind and therefore lower blood pressure and stress hormone production.

If you have already been diagnosed with heart disease, or if you've had a heart attack and wish to make a critical difference in your future prospects, it is recommended that you lower your intake of fat to 10 to 12 percent of your daily caloric intake. This involves some serious strategies for shopping, cooking, and eating. This diet prohibits any form of saturated fat. That means you should not consume anything that flies, swims, walks, or crawls—or any of their by-products.

A **very restricted low-fat diet** means no meats or organ meats, chicken, fish, processed deli meats, whole eggs or egg yolks, lard, suet, candy, store-bought baked goods, nuts, butter, margarine, sour cream, whipped cream, milk (except for skim), or other dairy products except plain, nonfat yogurt. You may occasionally use a small amount of canola or olive oil to saute vegetables or as a base for salad dressing.

The goal of the Ornish plan is to *reverse* heart disease—and in fact the statistics are so good that several insurance companies have agreed to reimburse patients for this type of treatment.

THE MIDCOURSE REHAB PLAN

Not everyone is emotionally equipped to make the radical changes called for by the Ornish plan. Very few individuals have the willpower and endurance to stick with it for more than a year. Once they start feeling better, they cheat on their diet, skip the stress management, and slack off on exercise.

Are they to be blamed for not putting their heart first? The truth is that women in particular are very socially conscious individuals, and it is hard to be invited to a barbecue and just eat green salad when all those around you are indulging in ribs, hamburgers, and potato salad. Do you act like a martyr and bring your own food with you wherever you go, risking the ridicule or pity of those who eat "normally"? Do you fall off the wagon just once a month for a special occasion and then get right back on it? Do you tell yourself you're feeling fine, and if you eat half of what everyone else at the party eats, you're still one up on them?

This is a difficult time in the life of a woman with heart disease.

Most of us are conditioned from earliest childhood to enjoy food for its taste rather than its merit as medicine. So at this late date, how do you substitute oat bran cakes for cookies? Collard greens for ice cream cones?

The sensible Midcourse Rehab Plan is followed by the second school of practitioners promoting heart health. If you can't throw out all the habits of the past, perhaps you can alter them favorably. If you are going to be miserable every time you walk into a supermarket or restaurant, the constant anxiety you feel may affect your heart. Making daily food choices that are abhorrent to you creates stress, and stress, as we know, damages your heart. Lean meat, fish, or turkey without the skin once a week may give you just the taste of your past that you crave.

The way that we interpret what food means in our lives is engrained—it comes to us when we are too young to understand its importance. For this reason diets constantly fail—even when the dieter knows that her life may be at stake. But the other aspect of healthy recuperation—exercise and stress management—don't appear to have the same emotional ramifications. Even if you hate exercise and loathed gym as a child, you can persuade yourself to take a walk in the morning air or around the mall. You can convince yourself that half an hour of quiet with the phone off the hook and nothing on your mind while you sit in the sun with your cat is relaxing and enjoyable.

The point of healthy eating, exercising, and mind-calming is to extend your time on earth so that you can do the things you want. It is not intended as a punishment or retribution for your former sins as a fat-eating couch potato. Therefore, you must find your own way to make this new lifestyle completely yours. If the plan you select comes to feel like part of you, you'll do it every day. If it feels alien, you'll never stick to it.

Look at the following options on your Midcourse Rehab Plan and pick the items that work for you right now, giving some consideration to those you'll add later on. You can start by selecting one new element a week, so that by the time you've been on the plan for three weeks, you'll be halfway into a new way of living. At the end of six weeks, you will be mixing and matching elements from each of the six categories every day.

The Midcourse Rehab Plan

WEEK ONE

Diet: Plant-based diet with two meat meals. One sweet, low-fat dessert every other day such as a lemon mousse made with egg whites or low-fat frozen yogurt.

Exercise: Daily fifteen-minute walk.

Stress: Daily fifteen-minute meditation or prayer.

Sleep: Daily, seven hours.

Smoking: If you are currently a smoker, search for a program, cut down to four cigarettes a day.

Drugs and Alcohol: Reduce alcohol to two ounces daily, eliminate any recreational drugs.

WEEK TWO

Diet: Plant-based, except for one restaurant meal where you may select liberally from pasta, lean meat, fish, or chicken cooked without butter.

Exercise: Daily twenty-minute walk, bike ride, or swim.

Stress: Daily fifteen-minute meditation, prayer, or one classical or jazz concert.

Sleep: Daily, seven hours.

Smoking: Begin program, cut down to two cigarettes a day.

Drugs and Alcohol: Reduce alcohol to two ounces every other day, eliminate any recreational drugs.

WEEK THREE

Diet: Plant-based, except for one meal, whether at home or out, where you may liberally select from pasta, lean meat, fish, or chicken cooked without butter.

Exercise: Half-hour daily of walking, biking, racquet sports, dance, etc.

Stress: Daily fifteen-minute meditation or prayer, consideration of joining support group or yoga or tai chi class.

Sleep: Daily, seven hours.

Smoking: Eliminate all cigarettes, continue program.

Drugs and Alcohol: Alcohol, two ounces every three days, no recreational drugs.

WEEKS FOUR TO SIX

Continue week three regimen and forgive yourself if you don't adhere to it every minute of every day. We all reach a plateau during behavior change. Just keep reminding yourself that this is a lifetime plan, and you have plenty of time to make it your own.

Reclaiming Your Sexuality

Is there sex after a heart attack? Of course there is! But only if you want it and spend a little time alone and with your partner learning what your new needs are and how to achieve them.

The stories of older men having heart attacks and collapsing over younger partners are legendary, and they spark all kinds of concerns in both partners about the advisability of getting too excited and exerting yourself too much. We don't hear stories of older women being rushed to emergency rooms by younger men partners—and this is a pretty telling omission in itself. It is difficult in our society for a postmenopausal woman to think of herself as sexy and desirable, let alone act sexual. There just aren't that many who have the self-confidence and eagerness to woo or be wooed by a younger partner.

But this is not to say that you can't or shouldn't be enthusiastic about your sexuality. Whether you have a long-term partner or are venturing into a new relationship, there's no reason to expect that you have to be abstinent after a cardiac event.

About four to six weeks after a heart attack, and usually the same period of time after heart surgery, you'll probably have recouped most of your strength and will be eager to get on with

your life. (If you've just had a catheterization or balloon procedure, you need only postpone sex for a day, while your puncture
wound heals.) If you're back to near normal at work and at
home, you can be sexual too. The point is how you relate to
yourself as a sexual being—and then, how your partner relates.

The bottom line is this: if you can walk up two flights of stairs
without panting and puffing, you can engage in sexual activity
and have an orgasm, or multiple orgasms. Sex is not that
strenuous—a woman's heart rate may rise from a normal of 80
beats per minute to 150 when she's in the throes of orgasm, but
it could easily rise to 130 just trudging upstairs. Also, remember
that this rise is brief and is not damaging to the heart. Nor is the
temporary rise in blood pressure, which is normal during the
flush of sexual excitement.

Once the peak is passed, and you and your partner are relaxed
together, the pulse rate and blood pressure drop—if you are
going to feel any palpitations or angina, it would happen at this
stage. Call your physician if you have heart palpitations that last
longer than fifteen minutes after sex, or if you're having any
difficulty breathing.

However, if you're fit enough to get up and down those stairs
mentioned earlier, we'll assume this probably won't happen.
Since you are undoubtedly enrolled in a monitored aerobic
program, your heart's capacity for sexual activity will increase as
you become more fit.

Finding Your Path Back to a Sexual Life

Sexuality includes a huge range of behavior. Only one tiny
portion of it is sexual intercourse. One of the best things about
recovery from a serious illness is that you know you are cherished
by your loved ones—and this is exactly the feeling you should
have before you consider a sexual encounter.

Many women are terrified of resuming a sexual life after a
heart attack or bypass surgery. They may be scared that an

orgasm will bring on another attack, or they may have deep-seated anxieties about their illness which, for many, cancels out the notion of being attractive and sexy. These fears are natural and normal, particularly right after a cardiac event, and you and your partner can simply go slowly together, relearning how important the power of touch can be between a couple. If you don't want to have intercourse initially, let your partner know. There are plenty of other intimate activities in which to indulge.

You can hug and cuddle, touch and kiss. You can partly undress your partner and give him or her a massage. You can take some spreadable foods into the bedroom and have a picnic on your partner's body. And he or she can do the same to you. You can spend hours delighting in each other's bodies and minds without ever touching the genitals. And you may or may not have an orgasm—it is certainly not a requirement.

On the other hand, if you are eager to celebrate life and want to launch into your sexuality with abandon, be sure to share that information, too! Many women, particularly after a serious illness, crave the sense of completion that intercourse affords. Sex after heart disease can be a slow and delicious build to a new bonding between you, and the physical connection you have with each other can cement the emotional connection. After all, if you care deeply for each other, you are inside each other's heart and soul anyway. And that's about as good as it can get.

In order to get back into a sexual relationship or enhance the one you had before you became ill, these are the steps you must take.

TALK

The two of you must come to some accord with the fact that things have changed. No one likes to admit it; people who've undergone traumatic events always want everything to shift back to just the way it was before, but this is impossible.

If you really communicated your sexual needs and desires before, you will not have too much difficulty expressing new thoughts and feelings now. If, however, you never talked together, this will be a whole new world for you—a little scary, but well worth the time and effort.

Make a time to talk that is not directly related to the bedroom—a long car trip is one option, or you can take each other out to lunch, either on the back porch or in a nice restaurant. Start with your feelings for each other and work your way up to the doubts and fears you may have about getting back to a sexual relationship. Tell each other (you may have to whisper if you're in public) all the things you'd like to do together. This can create the atmosphere for a very exciting encounter to come.

CONVINCING YOUR PARTNER IT IS OKAY

It is common to be scared about being sexual again after a heart attack, but some women are eager to have the opportunity to feel really alive and make love once again. What you do with your partner doesn't have to be strenuous or aerobic at first—you don't want to exhaust yourself with sexual pyrotechnics while you're recuperating. Both you and your partner will undoubtedly want to wean yourself back to this experience, both physically and emotionally.

Even if you're supremely confident about your sexual potential, your partner may need some convincing. Even though you may feel loving and want to get back into being a couple again, your partner may shy away. It will be up to you to set the mood and tone and assure your spouse that you're feeling fine and you really want to.

TAKE CHARGE

You get to decide whether or not you want sex, how much you want, when you want it, and how you want it. If you haven't been sexually assertive in the past, this is the time to start. It is so important for women to take charge of their sexual pleasure, and particularly so after a heart attack or heart surgery. When you ask for a little more time, a little more tenderness, a little more excitement, this adds to your partner's commitment to making this a joint activity. Sex can never be pleasurable or fulfilling when one person is *doing* something to another—even if it is meant well. Only when you participate in this adventure together will it really add something to your life.

DISCUSS ALL YOUR NEEDS, DESIRES, AND APPREHENSIONS WITH YOUR DOCTOR
You should, of course, discuss resuming your sex life with your physician. Remember, though, that many doctors aren't trained in sex therapy and might be more embarrassed about discussing the subject than you. If you find you're getting short shrift, there are professionals who specialize in recuperative sex therapy.

Another subject you should discuss with your doctor is hormone replacement therapy (see Chapter 6). Estrogen replacement can make a big difference in your comfort level, since the vaginal tissues respond and lubricate under the influence of this hormone. A Consumers Union survey on people over sixty showed that 93 percent of women on ERT or HRT were sexually active, as compared with 80 percent of women not taking replacement hormones. Also, if you are experiencing a loss of libido, you might want to consider taking Estratest, the medication that mixes estrogen with testosterone (the male hormone that helps with arousal and desire).

STOCK UP ON LUBRICANTS
You do not have to be postmenopausal to use a lubricant. As a matter of fact, a water-based product that gives a nice, slippery feeling can enhance the eroticism of any couple's encounters and make them all the more delicious.

After any serious illness or injury, as the body is healing, it is less likely to lubricate and stay lubricated for any significant time. And if you're nervous about having sex again after a long hiatus, you probably won't feel wet and aroused immediately.

Your local drugstore carries the ubiquitous K-Y Jelly (Johnson

& Johnson), but if this feels and smells too much like the gynecologist's office, there are a variety of new water-based products to try out. (*Never* use petroleum-based lubricants like baby oil, lard, butter, or hand lotion. They can damage fragile tissues and will also destroy any latex—a condom or dental dam—you may be using for safer sex purposes.)
Some of the newer lubricants are:

- Replens (Warner-Lambert)
- Astroglide (Biofilm)
- GyneMoistrin (Schering-Plough HealthCare)
- Lubrin (Upsher-Smith)
- Today Personal Lubricant (Whitehall)

MAKE UP A FANTASY

Sex is not a body-centered activity; the brain must first register desire, and a variety of hormonal and neural responses must encourage arousal before the genitals get into the act. So *thinking* about sex can make you sexier—and your imagination has unlimited potential.

Fantasizing is a wonderful way to get back to the closeness and intimacy you enjoyed before your heart attack or to inspire a new type of bonding that you've never had before. Fantasies may flit across your mind like daydreams, or they may be elaborate and involved with many settings, incidents, people, animals—whatever.

The easiest prescription for fantasizing is to recall a lovely incident from your past and conjure up all the details—how you both looked, what you were doing, where the furniture was, how the flowers smelled, how the birds sang. Take this experience and embellish it as you will, or leave it just as it was if it excited you.

Fantasies can also be wild and free and set a scene for something you would probably never want to happen in real life. You can imagine yourself naked under a waterfall with five partners about to make love to you if you wish—the idea is simply to allow your most incredible dreams to turn you on. After that, you can proceed to real life with a real partner.

DO SENSATE FOCUS/SHARING EXERCISES

Be sensitive to each other's new needs—and old ones. You may have to moderate the kind of activity you used to engage in, or change around elements of it. But this can be great fun! If you both enter into your sexuality with a spirit of adventure, you may find that sex is more rewarding to you than it was prior to your illness. The brush with mortality that you had can emphasize how much there is to be joyful about.

Here are some helpful hints that will help as you get back to a comfortable—and exciting—sex life.

1. Don't have sex after a heavy meal—your heart will direct more blood flow to the stomach to aid in digestion at that time.

2. Restrict alcohol consumption to two ounces a day. A little red wine is good for your heart (see Chapter 3), but an excess, particularly prior to a sexual encounter, will open the blood vessels too rapidly. Recreational drugs such as cocaine, marijuana, and amyl nitrate (poppers) are dangerous for people with normal hearts and could be fatal for someone with heart disease because they rapidly increase the heart rate.

3. Don't indulge in extremes of temperature before having sex—a sauna with a cold shower after it will cause a change in blood pressure as the blood vessels rapidly open and close. Even a hot bath can be dangerous right before sex.

4. Avoid positions where you're up on your arms a lot. Side-to-side positions are best.

5. Anal intercourse may lead to a slower-than-normal heart rhythm, which could be dangerous. Discuss this practice with your doctor before you engage in it.

6. If you are on high blood pressure medication, your libido may not be as strong as you would like. You might speak with your doctor about trying a different medication or a lower dosage.

What to Do to Avoid Another Heart Attack

A heart attack is a terrifying event, and it can cripple more than your blood vessels and heart muscle. Many people feel that they have a time bomb ticking inside them even months after recovery. They are just waiting for it to happen again.

The problem of the self-fulfilling prophecy ("If I believe it is going to happen, it really will,") is something we're going to work on right now. The following **ten-stage program** is designed to keep you from repeating that terrible trauma you already experienced and setting you on the road to a much more self-aware, healthier existence.

1. Give Up Your Give-up Attitude. Yes, you've been very sick, and you now know exactly what kind of condition your heart was in before it broke down. It is all too easy to sit back and allow the forces that caused your first heart attack to build up again.

If your primary risk factor was genetic, it will be hard to change the attitude that you might as well enjoy today because you're so unsure about seeing tomorrow. And yet it has clearly been documented that those who are observant in their lifestyle changes can alter if not reverse a predisposition to heart disease.

But you must never give up. The point of recuperating from a heart attack is to take yourself beyond healing the wounded body into becoming a truly healthy person. This will require a big shift in attitude. If you think you can be better than you were before your heart attack, you are well on the way to preventing a recurrence.

2. Work on Your Program Daily. The twelve-step programs have a maxim that goes, "It works if you work it." This means that you will only derive benefit from your ten-stage program if you conscientiously make it a part of your daily life.

3. Get into Rehab and Keep It Up After the Initial Months Are Over. Your physician will give you a prescription for two or three months in cardiac rehabilitation, where you will receive counseling and instruction in each element of their program. You'll come into the hospital or outpatient center two or three times a week for about eight to twelve weeks, and will be trained on a variety of machines as you wear a Holter monitor or simply have your vital signs checked on an ECG while you exercise. Insurance generally covers this two-month period, but if you wish to continue—which I strongly recommend that you do—it will cost about thirty dollars a month for a once-a-week visit.

You can, of course, join an approved health club with an okay from your doctor, and here you will also benefit from being supervised by one of the instructors who is aware of your cardiac status.

The point is to rehabilitate not only your heart muscle but also your approach to getting out of the house and doing some structured physical activity. The rehab center or health club is a wonderful place to meet others who will identify with and understand what you've been through and where you are going. A positive social climate—being surrounded by people who can really empathize with your situation—can effect a whole different level of healing inside you.

4. Know Your Body. Your lack of knowledge or denial of what was going on prior to your heart attack might have precipitated the event itself. Ignorance in the realm of health care is no excuse for getting sick a second time. At this point, you should be familiar not just with the terminology of the heart—the arteries, veins, capillaries, valves, etc.—but also with how your various systems behave at rest and in motion. Learning how to take your heart rate will be essential as you begin an exercise program; finding out what your blood pressure is like when you're anxious and when you're calm will give you a good barometer of how you react to stress. Knowing when you're winded and when you just need a few more seconds to recuperate can tell you whether or not to go on with the exercise you've been doing or to ask to have it moderated in some fashion by your doctor or rehabilitation specialist.

Know thyself. This is going to keep you vital and aware until you're past your hundredth birthday.

5. Try One New Activity or Challenge Each Week. Recovering from a heart attack can be incredibly boring. The things you used to love to do may be too taxing or may have been responsbile for your illness in the first place. This means you will have to find other ways of keeping busy—at least temporarily and possibly for the long run.

If you have always longed to study a new language or a musical instrument, this is the time to start. If you enjoy writing, composing music, or doing artwork, this is the time to start. If others have time to spend with you, come up with a project you can accomplish together. You might want to form a committee to do something environmental, or to help the community.

If you think it is too hard to start over, think again. After all, if you don't make a fresh start, you're back where you were before you got sick, and that's not a desirable place to be. You can work your way toward the best health you've ever had by reclaiming areas of your life you never knew you missed.

6. Educate Yourself and Others. A little knowledge can give you the groundwork to gain even more knowledge. Now that you've been through a cardiac event, you are an expert. You can talk "heart-speak" as well as any professional, you understand the diagrams of the way you work inside and you know what you have to do to keep healthy from now on.

But that's not enough. If you've ever learned a musical instrument, you know that in order to reinforce what you've already gained, it is important to practice regularly and challenge yourself a little more each time.

You can do the same with your heart knowledge by setting up or joining a support group. Many hospitals already have established programs—if they don't, you can take the initiative and lobby their rehab or education departments to start one.

You can also start a Heart-Wise group in your church, synagogue, or women's group. Many women who've had a heart attack or bypass surgery feel that passing on life-preserving information to others is now part of their job. It can be wonderfully supportive to gather together women who are currently in excellent health, women who are being medically managed for heart disease, and women who perhaps have been in denial about symptoms and should see a doctor. Passing information back and forth can be a real eye-opener—and it is always helpful to hear what it's really like from someone who's been there.

Another benefit of having a support group is that you can invite guest speakers. Cardiologists, internists, cardiac rehab nurses, respiratory and physical therapists are all usually willing to participate in these groups. And this way, more women who need referrals to good medical care can meet the practitioners "up close and personal."

7. See Your Physician at the First Sign of Pain or Difficulty. Just as managing a healthy heart is a team effort, so is preventing a second heart attack. Your team (see Chapter 9) is not disbanded just because your cardiac status has changed. Your primary physician will of course be expecting to see you every six months or so. But now, since you know your body so well, you will be able to identify any problems that should be attended to by other professionals.

Take all your medications in their appropriate dosages. If you find that you are having any unpleasant side effects (a lessening of libido with hypertension medication, for example), talk frankly with your doctor about changing dosages or changing the brand or type of drugs. *Never* stop taking a medication because it is too much trouble, or you think it isn't doing you any good.

8. Change Your Work Levels — or Your Work. You may feel that the best thing you can do after recovering from a heart attack is to get right back into the swing of things—and you may be absolutely right. It can be enormously beneficial to return to a comfortable routine, to life just the way we used to know it before we got sick. However, many of us suffer from jobs that sap our strength and energy without giving back a lot of creative juice. If this is your situation, you must make a change.

Whether you work for a large corporation or a small business, flextime is an increasingly popular way of managing staff. Have a serious discussion with your supervisor about changing or reducing your hours, or about doing a good portion of your work from home. If you run your own business, you are both in a less and more advantageous situation. On the one hand, only you know what is best for your business, and anyone else running it will naturally give it a different flavor. On the other hand, you have the ability to hire the people you need to take some of the burden off your back. You can restructure your own situation so as to give yourself ultimate control while passing the detail work onto others.

Finally, you may have a job that has burned you out and eaten you alive. Take this golden opportunity to stop doing what undoubtedly helped to produce the heart attack. Most companies are pretty liberal when it comes to sick leave, and you may be able to collect a year at partial pay with full benefits. During that time, you have the leisure to consider what you would like to do for the rest of your life.

9. Discover the Positive Effects of Laughter. This may sound strange, and even impossible, given your current situation, but documented evidence suggests that a cosmic sense of humor can actually heal the body as it soothes the mind. Norman Cousins, author of *Anatomy of an Illness,* explains that when he was diagnosed with a life-threatening disease, he went out and rented all the Marx Brothers' movies. He watched them over and over, laughing until the tears ran down his face. And in fact, the positive effect of concentrating on feeling good actually made a difference in his recovery.

If you can stand back and get perspective on your situation and laugh at your own frailties, fears, and weaknesses, you will be doing yourself an enormous favor.

10. Consider Psychological Counseling or Therapy. If you feel terribly fragile, and it is logical that you might, you may profit greatly from professional help. There is no point in living in fear. If you feel worried all the time that what happened before may recur, you may be brewing another cardiac episode or leaving yourself open to other illnesses and ailments. It is terrifying to relive the events of your heart attack and to contemplate what might happen if you had another, but if you cannot put these fears behind you, there are people who can help. It is quite common for cardiologists to refer their patients to a therapist or counselor right after a heart attack, but sometimes the effect doesn't take hold until later.

It is not your fault if you can't handle this alone. You're not expected to be an all-powerful woman with every inner resource. We are generally able to put the past behind us and go on with our lives only if we feel that there is no threat hanging over us. Therapy can make sense of the pressure so many feel after a heart attack and offer different emotional tools to help us proceed into the future.

Rebounding Back

It is painful for an adult to be reduced to the state of a dependent toddler. It is probably more painful for women, who are traditionally the strong ones, the mothers and wives and helpmates who do it all themselves. In addition to anticlotting drugs and specialized physical therapy, it takes guts and a sense of humor and complete faith in your own human spirit in order to heal from a heart attack or stroke.

When life has dealt some mean blows, the only way to cope is to fight back and keep fighting. In the next chapter, we'll learn exactly how to keep this positive force throughout our lives, through sickness and health.

12

Looking at the Rest of Your Life

∇

What do you want out of life? Are you content to continue as you have been, or are you ready to challenge the familiar and take some steps to make real change?

The answer to this question undoubtedly depends on whether you have yet had a brush with pain or disease. Usually, if we're feeling fine, we see no reason to make alterations in our comfortable patterns and routines. But if we've been in a difficult place and come back stronger, we know we can't simply allow life to carry us along blindly from day to day. Instead, *we* must carry life. We must take charge.

The Four-Facet Program for Revitalizing Your Life and Reducing Your Risk

You know that getting into good physical health and staying there is now your number-one priority. But how are you going to do this?

1. Nourishment. You must dedicate yourself to changing your attitude about what you put into your body. Learning to shop and cook and eat out and even go on vacation should be an ongoing project for you. This doesn't have to be an odious task—rather it should be a way of exploring new cuisines and new methods of nourishing your body. Buy some new cookbooks; take a course; spend time with friends who are also concerned with their good health.

"Cheating" never nets you anything, and can, in fact, be extremely dangerous. This is not to say that you shouldn't allow yourself liberal choices in your meals—however you know what's bad and what's good for you (if you don't, review Chapter 4), and it is stupid to try and fool yourself into believing that you're sticking to a health plan when you're not.

If you change your mind about what tastes good to you, you've won the battle. Only by experimenting with many different choices from the food pyramid will you learn how to enjoy the flavors and the benefits that really good nourishment can offer.

Change a little at a time—don't revamp your whole diet overnight. The incremental alterations you make in your eating habits will add up to a totally different way of approaching what you put inside you and how that affects your heart.

2. Exercise. Your program has to include *daily activity*, no matter what. Make it a point, when you start thinking about what you're going to do, to plan contingencies. If you love walking but live in a climate where you battle snowstorms or mudslides part of the year, do your two miles daily inside when you have to. Many malls around the country sponsor mall-walking clubs, which makes exercise a social as well as a physical event.

Vary your activities and you'll never be bored. You can walk and swim, bike and dance, play racquet sports and do tai chi. The body will thank you for cross-training by becoming more responsive and flexible. See Chapter 5 for more alternatives.

Motivation to exercise, just like motivation to stick to the right kinds of food, will not come overnight. If you have a setback—such as a bout of flu or back pain—don't let it stop you from thinking about exercise. Studies have shown that athletes who practice and also visualize doing well in their sport actually perform better than athletes who just practice. If you can motivate yourself to spend time each day just imagining a lovely jog on a country road, you will advance faster in your exercise program. Thinking about being active when you're not means you're more committed to an exercise plan even when you're inactive.

3. Stress Reduction. People have as many ways of reducing stress as they have ways of getting stressed out. The key, again, is to concentrate on what you want to get out of this program.

To reduce stress, you must acknowledge that you have it in the first place. This means taking an honest appraisal of your life and the difficult parts of it. You should know if you're stressed because of the knot in your stomach, the tension in your neck, the difficulty sleeping, the adaptive behavior that may involve drug, cigarette, or alcohol abuse.

You cannot become relaxed if you deny the concerns and anxiety that regularly push your buttons. Once you've mastered the job of identifying your stresses, you can start to tackle them. As we know from Chapter 5, ways to get rid of stress are exceptionally individual, but one of them is bound to work for you if you persevere.

4. Appreciation of Yourself. It's hard for many of us to admit we did something right—it is much easier to be self-critical and take the blame for everything. But until we start to appreciate what we uniquely provide for ourselves and others, we can never achieve real health. This is not just a catchall "feel-good" suggestion—it has actual ramifications in the way that we take care of ourselves. If we think there's something good there, we will eat better, exercise more, and spend more time relaxed than stressed. We will see our health-care provider when we should and stop denying that symptoms will go away if we just close our eyes and keep working.

Learn to like yourself. It is the best way to make sure that you pay attention to the preventive care details that can save your life.

Finding Out What You Want

Ask anyone you know what she really wants, deep down, and most will shrug. Do you want fame and fortune? Do you want a trip to Paris? Do you want to live to see your great-grandchildren? What about all of the above?

It is virtually impossible to strive for enormous riches or a Nobel Prize. Once you've decided that you *must* have certain things, you're sunk, because you've narrowed your goals, and you forget about all the other possibilities out there. You'll also end up bitter and disappointed if you don't get exactly what you feel you're entitled to. A more prudent tack is to begin with a few small things we know we can have, if we make some changes in our life. Those first steps will inevitably lead to bigger changes down the line, which should in turn lead to more positive results.

But the attitude comes first. What do you really want? Maybe it is better to start with what you don't want. Tell yourself in no uncertain terms:

- I resolve not to ignore any symptoms, no matter how small.
- I resolve not to accept poor treatment from any medical professional.
- I resolve not to be sickly and weak.
- I resolve not to be lonely, though I may be alone.
- I resolve that I will pay attention to my real needs and take steps to satisfy them.

Now that you are somewhat clearer on the negatives, let's tackle the positives. These will, of course, be different for every reader, and yet they'll have similar themes. Most individuals are looking for:

- a comfortable lifestyle
- good health
- a sense of inner peace
- real connection to others.

Although these positives may seem pretty vague, they are at least a start and correspond to what we've been saying right along about the holistic perspective—the factors that keep us in good heart health are many and varied and don't all relate to cholesterol or estrogen. We need more than all the preventive-care tactics we know we must implement. It is important for us to pay attention to the balance in our lives because it can be thrown off so easily without our knowledge.

If we lack that emotional part, that feeling that we have in some way succeeded in setting and achieving certain goals, we may not have the stamina to stick to a diet and exercise program. If we haven't made a true connection to others, we may not feel at home in a world that is often isolating and alienating.

The most crucial connection, however, is the one we make with ourselves. We have to care enough to make some goals, to reevaluate our behavior if it has been self-destructive or unprofitable. We need to connect with our true desires and find ways to achieve them.

Reevaluating the Caregiver Role

You probably can't count on your fingers all the responsibilities you have to others. Part of what makes most women thrive is the feeling that they're needed, that someone—that *many some-ones*—are depending on them daily. In fact, many studies have shown that the caregiver role is essential to women's survival, particularly in advanced old age. If nobody needs anything from us, if we don't provide some support to others, what are we here for? It is nourishing and uplifting to be there for those who rely on us.

However, we can easily go overboard with the caregiver role, and this is where a lot of women get into trouble. If you are responsible for a partner, a household, children (whether in or out of the house), elderly parents, a boss, several volunteer organizations, possibly a community or church group, and then you add a few pets, you are working full-time—overtime—for an incredible number of individuals. When do you ever get a chance to do something for yourself?

Little girls are taught from our earliest years to be generous and giving. The focus of Scouting and community service activities is teaching altruism and to love the other as yourself. And these are wonderful values to grow up with, except that many women carry them to ridiculous extremes.

Let us take the case of Rose, whom we met in Chapter 9. Even after she'd had a heart attack, she was determined to deliver all her Christmas presents before she would allow anyone to take her to the hospital.

It must be clear that Rose—and so many women like her, possibly even yourself—feel that they either don't deserve to be taken care of or simply haven't the time to be sick, so they tell themselves they're always well. When you refuse to admit that something might be wrong, you can't take care of it. This is called denial.

You've probably heard this term used in connection with people who have addictive problems—those who maintain that they could stop drinking or taking drugs if they chose or if they had a problem. Denying that anything is really going on when it is painfully obvious to everyone else is a big roadblock to health. And it isn't just the alcoholic or drug addict who denies his or her condition—it is an all-too-common problem for women with heart disease.

There are actually several levels of denial for the chronic caregiver who can't admit she needs help herself. The first level is a total rejection of symptoms and a seemingly careless attitude toward good preventive health care. The woman who's been having angina for years and persists in a diet of Big Macs and fried clams while protesting that she never has enough time to start a walking program is in denial.

A second level of denial occurs when her condition has progressed, even if it hasn't been diagnosed. At this stage, she undoubtedly has some serious symptoms that trouble her, but she is simply too scared to face them. It is at this point that she is opening herself to the real possibility of a heart attack or long-term damage to the heart muscle that may not be repairable. Yet another level of denial takes place after a heart attack itself. It may seem impossible that people who claim to have felt an elephant sitting on the middle of their chest can also claim that they are perfectly well, but it happens every day. Women in particular are able to con themselves into the belief that it was "just an episode, nothing much," and it will pass.

Janice, whom we met early in the book, suffered a heart attack in the middle of the night, experiencing all the classic symptoms of crushing chest pain radiating down her left arm and into her jaw. However, not wishing to disturb anyone at three in the morning, she lay there in bed, nauseated, covered with sweat, and shaking. In the morning, when she was unable to get out of bed, she told her sons, who happened to be visiting, that she was a little under the weather. She remained in bed, feeling increasingly worse, for three days before her children demanded that she let them take her to the emergency room.

Are you a denier? Are you so wrapped up in the caregiver role that you cannot make time for yourself? It is crucial to start examining this portion of your personality that may be either sustaining the level of illness you're currently at or leaving you open for future problems.

The Flip Side: You Don't Have to Be Selfless to Have Heart Disease

Not every woman spends her life taking care of others. For those who have spent most of their lives working for themselves, and often, living on their own, the caregiver role may not pertain at all.

But women who are bound up with their own success and think mostly about what they have to do to get ahead may also be candidates for heart disease.

Let's look at Claudia, whom we met in Chapter 10. She was a

total workaholic, determined to rise in the ranks in a field that was not traditionally open to females. Even when she was being wheeled into the emergency room, all she could think about was preserving her position in the fire department and having others think well of her service. She realized during her recuperation that her priorities were totally out of sync with her life.

A woman who is always a step ahead of her own achievements is putting herself under incredible stress. She may be so riveted on making more money, getting a leg up in her career, getting everything she wants—sometimes at the expense of others—that she neglects her health as badly as a woman who gives her all to those around her.

The pressures of meeting your own impossible expectations can make you sick. So if it can be harmful to adopt the caregiver role and harmful to put yourself first, what's the healthiest course?

Gain Perspective on All Facets of Your Life

In any heart health program, the first elements are diet and exercise modification. But the third, and by no means the least important, is lifestyle. It will take a very organized, thoughtful approach for both caregivers and ambitious workaholics to make some significant changes. Let's break down the areas of work so that you can tackle them one at a time.

There are five facets of your health arena, and they are interdependent on one another. Each will need some fine-tuning, and as you begin working on one, you will find that others fall into line more quickly. Don't neglect any of these—as you work on these areas, you will find that they interact and intersect in your heart health.

1. PERSONAL
   - your physical well-being
   - your partner or spouse
   - your children

- your parents
- your siblings
- your friends

How do you feel in your body over time? When you wake in the morning with twinges, what do you do about them? How does your physical health affect the way you deal with others? How do you relate to these particular individuals who are crucial to your emotional well-being?

2. WORK
- your job
- your colleagues
- travel on business
- further education
- personal projects
- financial planning

Do the details of your work make you crazy? Do you become so wrapped up in them that you cannot think about yourself? When you set yourself a goal, how crucial is it to you that you achieve it? Do you feel rushed to get there, or are you willing to let it move at its own pace?

3. HOBBIES/AVOCATIONS
- your house
- community or church activities
- cooking
- sewing
- artwork
- music
- writing
- whatever else gives you pleasure

First, ask yourself if you have any hobbies. If not, why not? Most people will make time for something that they are passionate about, and delving into these areas can be very rewarding and relaxing. Of course, there are others who attack hobbies with the same ferocious intensity they apply to their work. If this is your pattern, it is time to change it.

4. PHYSICAL LIFE
  - daily exercise for strength and flexibility
  - nutrition
  - dance (alone or with a partner)
  - sports—running, swimming, racquet sports, biking, etc.
  - camping
  - physical labor (building a bookcase; painting a wall; constructing a brick walk or patio; designing a rock garden)
  - sexuality

Even if you have previously ignored your physical life, if you make a start, you will find that it can become a positive addiction. There are so many different ways to nourish your body and to move it in space. The better you eat and the more you move, the better it is for your heart. Movement and physical activity have a strong mental and emotional component—certainly one's sexual life is made up in equal part of the physical and emotional. Working on your body therefore becomes integral to working on your mind.

5. INNER-CENTERED GROWTH
  - sense of well-being
  - reading
  - thinking
  - prayer
  - meditation
  - mentoring others

The part of you that can't be seen or touched is probably the most vulnerable when it comes to strengthening your heart. No physician or laboratory report can document what inner peace can do to the heart muscle. Yet in reducing stress, we are producing balance and harmony in the system. If you can achieve greater calm and enjoyment of life, you will work harder at the more concrete levels of good heart health.

The areas of self-work may seem overwhelming, but realize that you are now much more aware and attuned to things that may have gone wrong up to now. To make alterations in any of the five areas, you will have to do the following:

1. Prioritize. Decide which problems and projects are absolutely essential, and work on those. Everything else can wait.

2. Give others credit for being competent. If you work like a dog to complete everyone else's work, pick up after them and worry about them as well, you are in effect saying that they can't manage on their own. Of course they can! Things may not be done as quickly as you would do them, or exactly the same way, but they'll get done.

3. Make others wait if what they need is not crucial. You will get to them in time and provide whatever help they need eventually.

4. Boost your own self-esteem. Find at least five things you do every day that are worthy of a pat on the back. Stop whatever you're doing to congratulate yourself for an excellent job, well done. You deserve this and probably owe yourself several years' worth of back credit.

5. Block in some private time for yourself each day. You may do anything you like with it—write letters, lie in a hammock in the shade, give yourself a facial, dream up a perfect vacation. Just make sure it is an undisturbed half hour during which you can concentrate solely on yourself.

6. Don't feel guilty! This is the hardest one of all. It will take a lot of reassurance to let yourself do what you want to do. But the guilt is an old habit, and the more you tell yourself that there is nothing wrong with taking care of your heart, but everything right with it, the better off you will be.

There is a middle ground between being a *selfless* caregiver and a *selfish* individual who feels pressured to put her own needs first all the time. The woman who is *self-filled* can take care of both herself and others. This is the quality that will help you to take charge of your health. There is no reason that you have to give up your old roles entirely; all you have to do is trim the corners on the time you give to others and to yourself. If you let yourself get sick, remember, all those people who depend on you will be left in the lurch. But if you learn to treat yourself well, you will be extending your good health to all those who know you.

Goal Planning: A New Way to See Your Future

It is usually not until we have experienced a major setback or trauma in our lives that we start thinking about the future. Will there *be* a future? Will it be something to look forward to or something to dread? How will physical limitations impinge on mental awareness? On a social life? Can you be a woman with heart disease and still enjoy each day as it comes, looking forward to the next?

A lot has to do with your definition of yourself. If you see yourself as a "sick person" because you've had a heart attack or been through bypass surgery, you are starting off with a big handicap. You start to categorize yourself as a person who can't do certain things, can't participate in certain activities, and sure enough, you become that person.

In goal planning, your job is to work with only positive, self-fulfilling prophecies. You must start to see yourself as a well individual endowed with a healthy heart. It may be a medicated or surgically altered heart, but so what? It is still working hard twenty-four hours a day.

When you have something to live for and look forward to, you want to get up in the morning. When Marjorie Stoneman Douglass, who had worked all her life to save the Everglades, was interviewed on her hundredth birthday, she explained that she was busier now than she ever had been. "When I was in my eighties," she told the reporter, "I had the leisure time to get up, make ten phone calls, write ten letters, to get people interested in my cause. But now, realistically, I don't have that much time left to me. I have to get up and make twenty calls and write twenty letters."

This attitude is one to emulate. If you have suffered a major cardiac event, you have dealt with the fear and doubt, you have considered your own mortality. You know perfectly well that in order to restore your life to normal and to achieve the harmony and balance you need, it is going to be necessary to work harder at those things you previously took for granted.

What you have to do now is assume that you are starting from a perspective of health that will sustain you as you plan ahead. You will need to make short-term, long-term, and very long-term plans. Open yourself to the idea of planning and enjoying your own adventure, and you will find that your scope of possibilities immediately widens.

- Make one-, five-, and ten-year plans.
- Do what you *really* want to do.
- Plan with contingencies (be sure your goals are flexible so that you can do them alone or with a partner, depending on your current and future marital status).
- Think up new tactics for old problems—don't dismiss strategies or ideas because you think they're just "not you."
- Take some positive risks.

Making these plans will not only stimulate your imagination and ease you back into the swing of things, they will also eliminate your fear of loneliness and depression and may be able to reduce regrets you might have about all the things you might have done or should have done before your cardiac event.

HOW TO MAKE YOUR CUSTOMIZED PLAN

1. Create a list of your real, true interests, whether or not you ever pursued them. If you always wanted to be on the stage, write it down. If you saw yourself building a log cabin in the woods, write it down. Don't be afraid of your desires.

2. Pick five items on the list that you can see yourself dealing with in some form or other in the next six months.

3. Modify these five so that they conform more with your idea of what you're capable of. If you saw yourself in your dreams as a rock star, you could change the goal to being a soloist in the church choir or perhaps the leader of a women's a cappella singing group.

4. Write down some ways to go about getting to this goal. Suppose you want to start a band. You could list names of friends who are also interested in music, you could contact a local music school, or put an ad in the paper for musicians.

5. Of the five choices, start work on the one that best suits this time of your life. If you're still recuperating or in the midst of cardiac rehab, you may want to select a goal that doesn't require too much exertion or running around. (This doesn't mean, however, that you might not do those things next year!)

6. Consider how you could expand this goal after a year, five years, or ten years. What would you have to do to make this passion of yours a realistic achievement over time?

What might some goals be? Other women who have done this customized planning have come up with an interesting list:

- Go back to school.
- Travel.
- Volunteer at the local hospital or library.
- Teach illiterate adults.
- Run for public office.
- Start a business in your home.
- Sew, quilt, knit, or make jewelry and sell at local fairs.

- Teach a class at a local adult evening school.
- Learn a new language.
- Learn to play an instrument.
- Join a committee in your hometown.
- Become a foster grandparent to a troubled child.
- Coach a girls' basketball/hockey/soccer team.

There is nothing you can't do if you put your mind to it and your back into it. This is not to say the road will be easy, but when you plan ahead, you can't turn back.

Make Sure You—and Other Women with Heart Disease—Are Heard

There is another compelling reason to become vigilant about your own health, and that is because it will make you more aware of other women's health. There is so much denial about women's heart disease by the medical establishment, the third-party payers, and worst—women themselves. Until it is made perfectly clear, from laboratory trials, years of research including women, and testimonials of those who've been through the fire and come out the other side, who will know? Who will care?

If you have a friend who doesn't exercise, make her take a walk with you.

If you have a friend who subsists on junk food, cook up a banquet of vegetables and grains for her and top it off with a luscious plate of exotic fresh fruit.

If you have a friend who is always burdened with tension, talk to her about ways to use her stress constructively.

If you have a friend whose parent or sibling has just died of a heart condition, persuade her to have a baseline ECG.

If you have a friend who has chest pains, tell her it is probably not indigestion and offer to take her to your cardiologist, quickly.

If you are in a position of power in any field, and you can influence public policy, do so in behalf of women's health. You can offer no finer gift than the consideration and respect due all of us. Each woman should be able to know that she will get care when she needs it, that the drugs she takes or procedures performed on her are safe, and that her aftercare and recuperation will give her the time to rethink options and learn what she can do to change her own lifestyle and perhaps change her destiny.

Your New Awareness: Heart Disease Management as a Life Choice

This is your time. From now on, you are going to take positive risks for a new chapter in your life so that you can live well and happily into advanced old age.

You might say you have no choice now except to be enthusiastic about your nutrition and exercise, to manage your stress and anxiety, and to learn everything you possibly can about the way all your internal mechanisms—physical, mental, emotional, and spiritual—combine to make you the person you are.

Jennifer says, "I was truly blessed. I could have died, but I had incredible good luck—my own body helped me. So I have to admire that body and never take it for granted."

Claudia says, "I have my priorities in order. It used to be, get ahead in my career and forget everything else. Now I say, screw the job. My list is first God, then me, then my family, then work."

Rose says, "You got to know your limits. You can't go running to the doctor for every little thing, but when you're sick, it's important to go. I really learned about myself from my doctor, and then I wanted to please her and get well. So in doing what she told me, I helped myself."

If you are truly committed to keeping your heart in the best shape possible for the rest of your life, you have to make a deeper commitment—and this is to yourself. There is no one else, no physician, no friend, no pastoral counselor, no therapist, who can fix the way that you run your life. And in fact if you think about "fixing" anything, you're not starting from the point we've established, which is to *become* more yourself, not radically alter the person you've been up to now.

People evolve, just as lower life-forms have. We learn over the years what's really important. The interesting thing about becoming someone with a healthy heart is that so many other factors change once you start working your ten-stage program. The lightness in your step, the lack of fatigue, the ability to breathe deeply, the improved level of fitness, the tone of your skin and muscles, the way you look in clothes—and smell, if you've been a smoker!—all these elements create a better you.

Women are known as the fair sex, but we haven't been fair to ourselves at all. We have neglected our hearts and sometimes our souls, allowing others' problems to take precedence. We have allowed unthinking professionals to ignore our very real physical symptoms. We have in many instances been shunted aside through our own devices—we took what we could get and were grateful for it.

But it is time for quiet resignation to become active involvement. There is so much we can do and encourage others to do for us in terms of our health care. And let this be our goal: for the steady beat of that ever-working pump to remind us of the way we connect up with an even bigger rhythm—that of the spinning earth itself.

Each woman's mind and spirit needs to be grounded in the way she lives. By taking care of your heart, you can heal your life. Start today.

13

Where to Go for Help

▽

Many organizations around the country have specialized information and resources you can use to improve your heart health. Most will be happy to send you free brochures and different types of information to help you in your quest for excellent, specialized health care.

National Organizations

American Heart Association
7272 Greenville Avenue
Dallas, TX 75231
214-373-6300

Information on the heart itself, as well as heart health care. This organization offers up-to-the-minute data on the latest in prevention, medication, procedures, and surgery.

Mended Hearts c/o AHA
7272 Greenville Avenue
Dallas, TX 75231
214-706-1442

Support groups for patients and families after heart attack and bypass.

National Heart, Lung and Blood Institute
9000 Rockville Pike
Bethesda, MD 20892
301-496-4236

Research organization, also offers a wealth of information about heart and lung function.

National Stroke Association
8480 E. Orchard Street, Suite 1000
Englewood, CO 80111-5015
1-800-367-1990

Public service and research, offering the latest information on stroke and care for stroke patients.

National Women's Health Network
1325 G Street, NW
Washington, DC 20005
202-347-1140

For a five-dollar fee, they will send a packet of resource materials on any health-care subject relating to women.

North American Menopause Society
c/o University Hospitals of Cleveland
Dept. of Ob/Gyn
2074 Abington Road
Cleveland, OH 44106
216-844-3334

The most up-to-date information about hormone replacement therapy and wellness care for women approaching and past menopause. They can also offer referrals of physicians who treat women in midlife.

Regional Centers

These centers all offer information and support, as well as news-letters, nutrition, exercise, and stress-reduction programs, cardiac rehabilitation, and referrals to local physicians. Some sponsor Heart-Wise programs in churches and community centers.

Minneapolis Heart Institute Foundation
920 E. 28th Street
Minneapolis, MN 55407
612-863-3979

Women's Heart Research Foundation
PO Box 7827
West Trenton, NJ 08628
609-771-8313

Women's Healthcare Center and Heart Institute
Heartwise for Women
St. Francis Medical Center
601 Hamilton Avenue
Trenton, NJ 08629-1986
609-599-5025

Nutrition

American Dietetic Association
216 W. Jackson Boulevard, Suite 800
Chicago, IL 60606
312-899-0040

Center for Science in the Public Interest
1501 16th Street, NW
Washington, DC 20036
202-332-9110

Both of these organizations can give you solid, basic nutrition information and will have specific dietary references for good heart health.

Exercise

American College of Sports Medicine
PO Box 1440
Indianapolis, IN 46206
317-637-9200

Free brochures recommending healthy exercise programs for those with chronic disease conditions.

Stress and Heart Disease

Stress Reduction Clinic
Department of Medicine
University of Massachusetts Medical Center
55 Lake Avenue North
Worcester, MA 01655-0267
508-856-1616

This outpatient clinic offers an eight-week course for those with a chronic or acute medical condition. Mindfulness meditation and hatha yoga are taught as the tools to allow the patient to control his or her stress.

American Self-Help Clearinghouse
St. Clares-Riverside Medical Center
25 Pocono Road
Denville, NJ 07834
201-625-7101

This clearinghouse can put you in touch with self-help groups specifically working for more support in the heart-health area.

TM Training/Stress Management Courses

Your local community college undoubtedly offers several different stress-reduction and/or meditation programs. This won't require a great expenditure of time or money, since you can usually start in a ten-week beginner course to see how you like it.

Smoking

Smoke-Enders
4455 E. Camelback Road, Suite D150
Phoenix, AZ 85018
1-800-828-4357

One of the most reputable smoking-cessation programs in the country, Smoke-Enders has helped countless numbers of addicted smokers to stop. By calling their number, you'll be referred to a seminar in your local area or begun on a self-start home program that uses tapes, workbooks, and the twenty-four-hour helpline. This behavioral program helps you quit by first lowering your daily nicotine consumption, then dealing with the situational and diet problems that have made cigarettes part of your life.

American Lung Association
1740 Broadway
New York, NY 10019-4374
1-800-LUNG USA

This organization is dedicated to education, community service, advocacy, and research. When you call, you'll be directed to a local chapter in your area that runs smoking-cessation clinics and also can give you information on better lung health.

Diabetes

American Diabetes Association
1660 Duke Street
Alexandria, VA 22314
703-549-1500

This group offers information on the causes and treatment of diabetes, as well as helpful nutritional pamphlets.

Holistic Health Care

> Rise Institute
> PO Box 2733
> Petaluma, CA 94973
> 707-765-2758

This educational organization offers courses, workshops, and seminars to help people cope with chronic disease. The physical, emotional, and spiritual approach of the healing is based on the work of Sri Eknath Easwaren, a meditation teacher who created a program of holistic healing.

> American Holistic Health Association
> PO Box 17400
> Anaheim, CA 92817
> 714-779-6152

This organization publishes information on holistic approach to health care.

> American Holistic Medical Association
> 4101 Lake Boone Trail, Suite 201
> Raleigh, NC 27607
> 919-787-5146

This group of physicians dedicated to holistic medical practices may offer referrals to doctors in your area who are members.

> Center for Mind-Body Studies
> 5225 Connecticut Avenue, NW, Suite 414
> Washington, DC 20015
> 202-966-7338

The Center provides education and information for anyone wishing to explore their capacity for self-care and self-healing. They also sponsor self-help groups for people with chronic illness.

Mind-Body Medical Institute
Mercy Hospital and Medical Center
Stevenson Expressway at King Drive
Chicago, IL 60616-2477
312-567-6700

This institute runs a cardiac risk modification program that integrates Western medical practice with behavioral therapy in order to reduce blood pressure, cholesterol level, and control diabetes. Mind and body techniques (including practice of the relaxation response) are taught to patients by an interdisciplinary staff.

Preventive Medicine Research Institute
900 Bridgeway, Suite 2
Sausalito, CA 94965
415-332-2525

This organization, founded and directed by Dr. Dean Ornish, offers training programs and conducts research in mind-body medicine.

Available Libraries and Databases

If you're on-line with any good computer network, such as Medline or Paperchase on Compuserve, you can look up articles from medical libraries all over the country. You may wish to read the abstracts on your screen and then have certain articles printed out or mailed to you for an extra fee.

Most medical school or hospital libraries are accessible to the general public, and you can request specialized information from the librarian. You may also wish to contact the groups below:

Center for Medical Consumers/Health Care Library
237 Thompson Street
New York, NY 10012
212-674-7105

This is an excellent resource for books and the latest articles on traditional and alternative medicine. They also publish a monthly newsletter called *Healthfacts*.

World Research Foundation
15300 Ventura Boulevard, Suite 405
Sherman Oaks, CA 91403
818-907-5483

This organization provides information packs on health subjects. For a fee of $45 plus shipping, they will research either standard or alternative medical approaches to any disease or condition, culling information from 5,000 medical journal articles and a variety of books on complementary treatments.

Planetree Health Resource Center
2040 Webster Street
San Francisco, CA 94115
415-923-3681

Planetree offers an In-Depth Health Information Packet for $100, which offers a selection of up-to-date medical references, or you can order a $20 bibliography of source materials. They can also supply you with their directory of physicians and other health-care practitioners, organizations, and support groups.

The Health Resource
Janice R. Guthrie
209 Katherine Drive
Conway, AR 72032
501-329-5272

Will provide reports on traditional and alternative treatments of specific medical problems for a fee of $195 plus shipping.

Newsletters

Harvard Heart Letter
Harvard Medical School Health Publication Group
PO Box 420234
Palm Court, FL 32142-0234

Thirty dollars a year for twelve issues.

Cardiac Alert
George Washington University Medical Center
Phillips Publishing Inc.
7811 Montrose Road
Potomac, MD 20854

Seventy-five dollars a year for twelve issues.

Diet-Heart Newsletter
PO Box 2039
Venice, CA 90294

Fifteen dollars a year, quarterly, published by health book author Robert Kowalski, including recipes and nutritional information.

Heartline
Cleveland Clinic Educational Foundation
Coronary Club, Inc.
9500 Euclid Avenue, E4-15
Cleveland, OH 44195-5058

Twenty-nine dollars a year for twelve issues.

Good Cooking

In order to keep your heart in good shape, you have to eat right. Here are some recommended heart-healthy cookbooks:

1. *The American Heart Association Cookbook,* 4th revised edition, David McKay Co., New York, 1986.
2. *The Gourmet Low Cholesterol Cookbook,* by Elizabeth Weiss and Rita Wolfson. Fore Paperbacks.
3. *Craig Claiborne's Gourmet Diet,* by Craig Claiborne. Ballantine Books, 1985, New York.
4. *Don't Eat Your Heart Out Cookbook,* by Joseph C. Piscatilla. Workman Publishing Co., Inc., NY, 1983.
5. *The New American Diet,* by Sonja L. Connor, M.S., R.D., and William E. Connor, M.D. Simon & Schuster, New York, 1989.
6. *Quick and Easy Recipes to Lower Your Cholesterol,* by Lori Longbotham. Avon Books, New York, 1989.

Recommended Reading

Benson, Herbert, *The Relaxation Response.* Morrow, New York, 1975.

Braiker, Harriet B., *The Type E Woman.* Dodd, Mead, New York, 1986.

Frankenhaeuser, Marianne, ed. *Women, Work, and Health.* Plenum Press, New York, 1991.

Goldman, Martin, M.D., *The Handbook of Heart Drugs.* Henry Holt, New York, 1992.

Hochman, Gloria, *Heart Bypass: What Every Patient Must Know.* St. Martins Press, New York, 1982.

Kabat-Zinn, Jon, *Full Catastrophe Living.* Delta Books, New York, 1990.

Kabat-Zinn, Jon, *Wherever You Go, There You Are.* Hyperion, New York, 1994.

Legato, Marianne J., M.D., and Carol Colman. *The Female Heart,* Avon Books, New York, 1991.

J. J. Lynch, *The Broken Heart.* Basic Books, New York, 1977.

———. *The Language of the Heart: The Body's Response to Human Dialogue.* Basic Books, New York, 1985.

Ornish, Dean, M.D., *Dr. Dean Ornish's Program for Reversing Heart Disease.* Random House, New York, 1990.

Pashkow, Frederic J., M.D., and Charlotte Libov. *The Woman's Heart Book.* E. P. Dutton, New York, 1993.

People's Medical Society. *Your Heart: Questions You Have, Answers You Need.* 1992.

Roth, Eli M., M.D., F.A.C.C., and Sandra L. Streicher, R.N. *Good Cholesterol, Bad Cholesterol.* Prima Publishing and Communications, 1990.

Samuels, Mike, M.D., and Nancy Samuels. *How to Work with Your Doctor and Take Charge of Your Health: Heart Disease.* Summit Books, New York, 1991.

Wolinsky, Harvey, M.D., and Gary Ferguson. *The Heart Attack Recovery Handbook.* Warner Books, New York, 1988.

Index

Italic page numbers indicate material in tables or illustrations.

ABOUT THE AUTHORS

ELIZABETH ROSS, M.D., F.A.C.C., is a cardiologist in private practice in Washington, DC, and a fellow of the American College of Cardiology. She is affiliated with Washington Heart at Washington Hospital Center and was the 1993 chairperson of the committee on women and heart disease of the Washington chapter of the American Heart Association. She is currently active in the organization's programs committee on women's health issues.

JUDITH SACHS has been a writer and speaker for the past fifteen years and is the author or coauthor of thirteen books about preventive health care. She conducts workshops on the topics of menopause, sexuality, and midlife change for several holistic centers, universities, and corporations and is an adjunct professor at Trenton State College in the Department of Health and Physical Education.